W9-AGT-162

Also by Serita Stevens

*Ten percent of the proceeds from these books will go to "Hugs and Hopes" in Romania.

FORENSIC NURSE

THE NEW ROLE OF
THE NURSE
IN LAW ENFORCEMENT

Serita Stevens, RN, BSN, MA, LNC

St. Martin's Paperbacks

Ten percent of this book's author proceeds go to an IAFN scholarship fund for nurses studying forensics.

Serita is now rewriting and assisting with the re-release of *Cherry Ames, Nurse Detective* and her new version of *Charlie London*. Royalties for these books go to nursing scholarships.

FORENSIC NURSE

ISBN: 0-312-35612-9
EAN: 9780312-35612-5

Printed in the United States of America

St. Martin's Press hardcover edition / September 2004
St. Martin's Paperbacks edition / August 2006

St. Martin's Paperbacks are published by St. Martin's Press, 175 Fifth Avenue, New York, NY 10010.

10 9 8 7 6 5 4 3 2 1

Our lives begin to end the day we become silent about the things that matter.

—MARTIN LUTHER KING JR.

Contents

FORENSIC
NURSE

Who Is a Forensic Nurse?

Saturday night. The bars are full. So is the emergency room. The usual suspects jam the cubicles, overflowing into the halls: a brawl victim with a broken hand; a baby with a high fever; a truck driver who complains of dizziness; a man, claiming to hear voices, who has stabbed his sister; the police are on their way in with the second of two rape victims and a DOA (dead on arrival).

Gunshot wounds, stabbings, and drug overdoses are common here, in this large metropolitan hospital.

One victim, a walk-in patient, is a young woman in a blood-spattered dress, bruises covering her face and body. She says she fell down a staircase in her home.

The admitting physician, an intern, interviews her briefly. Assisted by a nurse, he examines her and orders X-rays. He finds no life-threatening injuries but does observe evidence of earlier abrasions and contusions. Visibly upset and nervous, the patient explains them away, saying they were from tripping over her child's toy, and other household accidents. With at least a dozen patients waiting for him and ambulances bringing in more, the intern treats the woman's cuts and discharges her.

Is it possible that, under the pressure of a crushing caseload, he inadvertently released a victim of domestic violence without taking time for the appropriate follow-up?

Had the assisting nurse been a forensic nurse, there would have been little chance of that.

In fact, many patients in the emergency room have one thing in common: They are cases for the forensic nurse.

Any time a nurse treats a victim of a criminal act or someone suspected of committing one, the survivor of a catastrophic accident, or any other victim of a bodily injury, living or dead, where liability may be involved, she* is involved in a forensic case, one that requires investigation beyond the medical.

The forensic nurse (FN) is the new detective on the block. She is law enforcement's secret weapon. The expertise of a forensic nurse—a unique combination

---

*Author's note: Because it is still the case that most nurses are female, the pronoun "she" is used commonly throughout the book. Actually, however, there are also male nurses in the profession— and male victims of rape.

of medical skill, legal knowledge, and criminology—makes her input increasingly more valuable in the investigation of crimes. "Forensic nursing" is a relatively new term and has been formally accepted as a specific area of the nursing profession only recently, after it was recognized by the American Association of Nurses in 1996. Forensic nursing has quickly become one of the newest medical specialties, although nurses have been contributing to forensics for centuries.

Forensic nurses are the link between the health-care profession and the criminal-justice system. In most cases, their expertise is available at the point of first contact—the door to the emergency room.

Forensic nurses have been trained to identify the weapon consistent with the patient's injury; to interview victims in order to get the fullest and most accurate story; and to recognize, collect, and preserve evidence. They have developed the healthy skepticism that enables them to assess the validity of accounts from both victim and suspect. Such specialists are valuable liaisons between the law enforcement and the medical profession, and, unlike many medical professionals, they have the training and experience to testify effectively as expert or actual witnesses.

Like Molière's bourgeois gentleman surprised to learn that he has been speaking prose all his life, many in the profession have often served as forensic nurses in the course of their duties without being aware that they were doing just that. From the moment they first entered nursing school, they were warned that anything they did or said to or about the patient could wind up in court. (Back then, not many students looked forward to being relied on as expert witnesses. In fact, a nurse with a crime-related case was usually petrified at the prospect of being called to the witness stand and questioned about his or her abilities and competence.)

However, at that time, because there was no training in forensic care, nurses knew neither what it involved nor how they might contribute to lessening the crime and violence they encounter every day.

One of the definitions of "forensic" is "employed in or pertaining to the legal profession." Yet the term "forensic nurse" is still not understood by many. Growing up with TV's popular *Quincy*, who played the part of a forensic pathologist, many assumed the word meant "death" or "working with death." But forensic cases include the living as well as the dead. Anything that is a factor in a legal case can be called "forensic." This includes insurance cases and others where the law might be involved. Victims of rape, abuse, and trauma occupy one in every eight hospital beds. Every day six thousand violent crimes are committed or attempted in the United States (Reiss, 1993).

What I saw in the course of my usual nursing duties made me want to learn more about what a nurse could do when she or he encounters a possibly criminal situation. Stumbling across an e-mail address "SleuthRN," I contacted the person behind it to learn what that meant.

SleuthRN, aka Sandra Goldstein, is a sexual assault

nurse examiner (SANE) in Santa Cruz, California. When I reached her, she directed me to the International Association of Forensic Nurses (IAFN). That was when my working life took a fascinating turn.

Attending the organization's Third Scientific Assembly in Louisville, Kentucky, I learned what "forensic" meant as it applied to nursing. Forensic nurses are specialized nurses who fill a void in emergency rooms, where most doctors have little or no forensic training, which can often be a serious handicap. To counter it, the IAFN works to bring forensic nurses together with pathologists, criminologists, and others who can help them perfect their skills and widen their abilities. This organization is only a few years old, but it already has over a thousand members and is growing daily.

IAFN was founded in 1992 by seventy-four pioneers, spearheaded by Linda Ledray, Ph.D., who had started the Minneapolis sexual assault response team (SART). It was a step into an unknown territory. Linda had been writing about sexual assault examinations for the *Journal of Emergency Nursing*. She wanted to find out who else was out there performing sexual assault exams and how they were doing it. She wanted to know what successes they had, what failures, and why. The only way to grow was to learn from one another as a community. So, in the summer of 1992, she organized a meeting of nurses in Minneapolis. Most of those attending considered themselves SANE, since among their other duties they performed rape exams of both the victims and the perpetrators—when those were known. Nurses who attended found out that they were not alone in their quest for justice and their desire to see the victims properly taken care of and guided through the judicial system. One nurse described the experience as akin to "finding your long-lost best friend."

During this meeting, the nurses found out that although different groups had various routines for examining victims of rape and other trauma, they were unanimous in believing that there was a better way to help victims and survivors than the present practice. SANEs began to organize. There were bumps in the road, but they moved on. They braved the "old-boy network," stumbling and pushing forward with the courage of Florence Nightingale. They entered the realm of death investigation as nurse coroners or deputy coroners and earned the respect of their male colleagues. In Wisconsin and in Texas, nurses fought to use their medical and legal skills to assist the survivors of trauma as well as to carry out their forensic investigations. A large group took on the bar associations to become accepted as nurse-attorneys or nurse–legal consultants.

Yet no matter what they added to their nursing degrees, all of them remained nurses. The unique perspective provided by their nursing skills gave them a leg up in solving problems. Their training and abilities could help the victims in ways law enforcement had never contemplated. Their attitude towards the body as the crime scene took them places and provided them with key questions that no one without their training would ever think to ask.

Many crime victims are able to get to the emergency room on their own; consequently, when they arrive, they haven't even talked to the police yet. A high percentage of ER patients who need urgent care are forensic cases. Victims of rape, of felonious assault, and, of course, of homicide are obvious examples. But workman's compensation cases, accident liability, domestic violence, child abuse, elder abuse, food and drug tampering, automobile accidents, attempted suicide, and hazardous environmental contamination all come under the umbrella of the dictionary definition of "forensic."

Virginia Lynch, the former president of IAFN, says: "There are puzzles involved; it's up to the forensic nurse to identify what is going on, to listen to the silent language and put the pieces of that puzzle together.

"I went to the local crime lab," she says, "to find out what we could do to better protect the patient's legal rights and properly preserve evidence. Inside the lab, the door of forensic science opened. I realized that tremendous void exists between the health and justice systems. I saw that victims were often treated less than empathically by both law officials and health care professionals. They felt uncomfortable with the emotional trauma surrounding crime victims as well as their families, much of which, due to time constraints and lack of necessary skills, could not be addressed properly."

Lynch was determined to incorporate crisis intervention and grief counseling into these cases. This was a road to recovery that only a qualified nurse could help with. And hand in hand with the training for this went the special skill of forensic investigation.

Because of Virginia's efforts, word of the new specialty spread around the globe—to Canada, England, Japan, Singapore, Russia, and South Africa, where the murder rate is one of the highest in the world. Some Caribbean and Central American countries also joined the forensic nursing family.

Law enforcement took notice but not enough. The nurses' services and resources were still underused. Battles had to be fought. Turf wars broke out. But slowly—too slowly for us—things began to change. More hospitals began employing forensic nurses, and the nurses at more hospitals had at least some of the necessary training.

Despite that training, very few were awarded full-time positions for their efforts. Weeks would pass without a single day off. In the trauma center, where the usual procedure was "a shot, a Band-Aid, and thank-you-ma'am," the rest of the staff resented the SANEs and left them without support to do four- to six-hour forensic exams and evidence collection for rape victims. And they were further irritated when the SANE then had to be absent from work in order to appear in court.

Who was supposed to pay for those hours? Who was going to fund a SART station or stations? Hospitals? Law enforcement? Some centers obtained funding from projects such as Violence Against Women. Some received grants from the Department of Justice. But the money available was seldom enough for the state-of-the-art equipment needed and the cost of the nurses' time.

And then there were the doctors, too many of whom felt that the nurses were encroaching on their area. They were angered by the nurses' audacity to do pelvic exams or use the colposcope on their own. The colposcope, an instrument originally used for magnification of cells to identify vulval cancer, was later found to be an excellent aid in getting helpful photographs of such trauma as child abuse injuries. But the medical establishment seldom adopted its use on adult victims of sexual assault as a standard practice, even though there is no better way to differentiate forced sexual contact from consensual. Doctors have the medical knowledge needed to recognize the signs and symptoms of many diseases. They know how to tell physical abnormalities from the norm. But medical school never taught them to identify patterned injuries or to distinguish blunt from sharp-force trauma. That kind of information, however, is a significant factor in discovering what, and consequently who, is responsible for an injury. It is information that forensic nurses can provide and the doctors cannot.

It is assumed that doctors can treat trauma. They can. But very few of them understand the different treatment that *forensic* trauma requires. Their education does not include identifying wound patterns or some sexual injuries. They don't know how to collect evidence so that it will not be challenged in court. Some doctors, knowing that they lack the necessary proficiency to back up their evidence, often shy away from being called into court to be questioned by a hostile defense attorney. Many refuse to perform the medical-evidence exam. And many doctors, while flattered at being called expert witnesses, are not.

Doctors became upset when nurses who were not part of the hospital staff started being called in to do rape exams. Yet they were relieved not to have to deal with the courts. The average ER doctor has no training (or willingness), when it comes to doing a forensic exam or collecting evidence. In fact, doctors and untrained nurses frequently throw away or destroy evidence without recognizing its high importance. Overwhelmed by the sheer number of cases, especially in major trauma centers, they often simply do not have time to stop, to collect and preserve clothing, body fluids, and trace materials, all of which could be important evidence.

Very few medical and nursing schools in the United States and elsewhere teach forensic medicine. The few that do teach it only as an elective.

Frequently, even though the doctor or ER nurse knows what should be done, he or she will fear inadvertently violating the patient's confidentiality or constitutional rights and end up with a lawsuit on their hands.

The kind of investigation a forensic nurse is trained to

do is also indispensable in cases of questionable death. Pathologists can make great coroners and medical examiners, but there are too few around. Fewer than four hundred certified forensic pathologists practice in the United States and only a fraction of these are willing to do the work of the medical examiner. To fill the positions, many agencies have turned to nurses. Because nurses are trained to understand how the body functions, they can determine more quickly whether a death is natural or unnatural. They can tell if the medications the person had taken had hastened their death or did not affect it. They know when something looks suspicious and when it does not.

Dr. John Butts, chief medical examiner of the Canadian province of Alberta, adopted the practice of hiring forensic nurses as death investigators. He carried the practice with him to Nova Scotia when he relocated there. But this intelligent solution to the shortage of medical examiners has not been adopted in enough places in either Canada or the United States. Within the United States, only a handful of chief medical examiners have made the same discovery.

Many police, district attorneys, prosecutors, and judges do not know how to use this new weapon. In court, they still look to and expect expertise from the doctors rather than the nurses, in spite of the nurses' additional training and special skills in forensic exams. Bypassing nurses who have actually seen the wounds and can correctly identify them, law enforcement turned to the nearest doctor who may never before have encountered the entrance or exit wound a bullet makes. The mistaken answer the doctor may give often alters the whole course of a trial.

Seeing only the stereotype of women in starched white carrying a bedpan, the courts forget that the nurse, who has always been the liaison between the doctor and the public, is a skilled translator of medicalese. Teaching is one of the basic nursing skills. As a by-product of their nursing education, they are expert in educating and persuading a jury, not in medical jargon but in language the lay listener can understand.

Moreover, the public itself, unaware of these specially trained nurses and their potential in helping fight crime, does not seek them out or know that their advice could help make recovery from the grief and trauma much easier. Taught to use their knowledge and skills to treat the whole individual and to see the whole picture, forensic nurses often play the role of resource person—someone who can arrange the various disciplines or puzzle pieces into a recognizable whole that will help trauma victims to heal.

It is the nurses who are at the forefront of trauma treatment and death investigation. Nurses are almost always the first to see the victims as they are brought into the emergency room. But there are also nurses who work as an adjunct to the medical examiner. They investigate unnatural deaths, join the paramedics in triage, serve as consultants to lawyers and district attorneys in both criminal and civil cases. Some are nurse-attorneys themselves.

Often it is a nurse who photographs the evidence and notes the wound patterns, who works as a police liaison, and is the first to pick up signs of child abuse and domestic violence.

Forensic nurses who are part of a disaster medical emergency team (DMET) assist not only in providing medical resources to overwhelming numbers of victims in mass tragedies, but a disaster mortuary operations team (DMORT) can help to identify parts of bodies after lethal crashes and hurricanes.

Forensic nurses have served as expert witnesses in court, helping to get convictions by uncovering fraud and providing evidence, investigating work-related and vehicular accidents, and, in teamwork with the police, contributing to the solution of many cases of unnatural or suspected deaths. Armed with the knowledge needed to trace by ballistics, the source of gun wounds, to find out the details of a rape by examining the victim, and more, nurses in forensics have increased the odds that rapists and killers will be captured—and that the falsely accused will be exonerated.

The forensic nurse is someone who cares enough to be aware of both the medical and legal side of the exam; someone with a passion for justice, someone who wants to make a difference in people's lives.

Rampant violence and its consequences is a public health problem that needs addressing. Finding an effective answer to violence in America and the world at large requires cooperation among many disciplines.

Forensic nursing is contributing its particular skills to the solution of this worldwide problem.

IAFN's motto is "Nursing Beyond Tradition." "We nurses are no longer the bedpan pushers our mother Florence Nightingale was," says Diana. "While we still hold the patient's hand, and are concerned about the physical and emotional trauma the victims of forensic cases are suffering, we can also find ways to go beyond tradition and put a stop to the violence. Working together, nurses, doctors, law enforcement, science, and the public can make a difference in our lives and in our society."

Diana is one of the unsung heroines of IAFN. She helped with the original development of the group. "I get surprised when people tell me that I am one of the pioneers. It feels good that my name is known, but I didn't start doing this to break new ground."

Like most of us who have become hooked on forensic nursing, Diana read the early Cherry Ames novels* and realized that there was more to helping people than passing bedpans. "Everyone has their own niche. I could never be a CCU nurse, but forensics is my field."

As many other nurses, Diana credits forensics with turning her whole nursing career around. "It became more of a challenge to me," she says. Diana works with the American Academy of Forensic Science and is also active in establishing nationwide standards for the

*The series is being reissued. I am one of the writers.

SANE, often volunteering her time to chair various committees on ethics and protocol.

Originally a head nurse in a pediatric unit, she had helped put the child abuse program together in her home area. The local police were so pleased with the results and with how much easier the prosecution of their cases went that they asked if the hospital could put something together for adults who had been sexually assaulted. "We're tired of getting the runaround and of waiting for hours upon hours in the emergency room for a spot in the triage line," one cop told her.

And so the SART program was born in 1990 at Pomerado Hospital in San Diego.

One of the earlier groups, they were lucky to have Dr. Laura Slaughter, who pioneered some work on rape victims and evidence-collection, and Sherry Ardnt as their trainers.

"If you don't know something exists, you won't be looking for it. Now we see evidence in places we never would have thought of before," Diana says. "Until I was educated about the role of nursing in forensics, I was clueless about all the implications. Now I see clues everywhere, and it helps the police and the DA with the case investigation and prosecution."

Diana credits Virginia Lynch with the original article that defined forensic nursing. "I never would have put all that together the way she did. She included death, legal, child abuse, domestic violence, forensic psychiatry, trauma, workman's comp . . . all these areas that I wouldn't have thought of."

She admits that there are still a lot of obstacles for the forensic nurse to overcome. "One of the biggest issues is credibility," she says, "and helping the jury and judges to understand that we are nurses, not doctors, yet still recognize our advanced skills and experience. Most doctors have no training in courtroom testimony and really do not want to go to court. Forensic nurses are trained to do just that."

John became convinced of the value of medical-legal training when he heard Virginia Lynch, whom he had known in school years before, speak. He realized that forensic nursing was his calling. "I want to do something to help people. I get a lot of satisfaction out of it.

"Clinical forensics, which encompasses sexual assault, domestic violence, child abuse, work injuries, MVAs (motor vehicle accidents), has just about everything. I took sexual assault training, a medical-legal death investigation course, and I even did an internship at the coroner's office in Reno, Nevada.

"I watched Henry Lee testifying in court and I knew I wanted him to teach me blood-splatter analysis. One thing led to another, and soon I was giving lectures about forensic nursing, just like Virginia. I want to light fires under people and let them assist us with seeking justice."

John now teaches others how to recognize evidence and then how to preserve it. "Once we know that, we transport it correctly and use it to testify. All that makes law enforcement a lot easier." A large number of police and law enforcement personnel come to his classes, as well as nurses.

And then there's Jennifer. Nurses like Jennifer have a hard time getting established as forensic nurses because even though we do forensics in the emergency room daily, most people, even the nurse managers, and especially the doctors, don't see it as necessary.

She was forced to pay for the SANE training and other training that she has since taken on wounds and ballistics out of her own pocket, as have most of the nurses referred to in this book.

Only after the hospital administration saw how cost-effective it was to have a forensic nurse on duty, because, among other reasons, they no longer had to give doctors time off to go to court as often, and how her training gave the hospital bonus points with the community, did the hospital pay for other nurses to attend the courses.

"But it wasn't easy with police, either," Jennifer says. "We each had to feel our way. Building trust between the police, the doctors, and myself was a painstaking, often frustrating process. I couldn't just go up to them and say, 'Hi, I'm your new forensic nurse.'"

The police, Jennifer reported, were more receptive than the doctors because they stood to benefit the most—more perps arrested and easier collars for them.

The doctors were a different breed altogether. "On some level," she says, "they still remain a bit distant, despite the fact that they hate going to court, they hate getting called at two a.m. I love it." The presentation of observations has to be made at a more diplomatic level. "Doctor, did those bruises look suspicious to you? Do you think they were at different stages in healing?" Or "We often collect blood so we can rule out———. Shall I collect that for you?"

Diplomacy is essential, because most SANE programs have a policy requiring a patient with specific injuries or preexisting histories—such as genital bleeding, pregnancy, insertion of a foreign object, difficulty breathing, loss of consciousness, or being under fourteen years of age—to be seen by a physician before the nurse can do the SANE exam. It is only when a patient is not severely injured that the triage desk is bypassed. The SANE must always consult the attending physician regarding prophylactic antibiotics, pregnancy prevention, and other orders, before she develops a specific patient plan of care.

Despite the frustrations, Jennifer and the others who work ER trauma forensics report that when a case is won, "it's the best possible high." Not only that, when a case is won, and the proper credit is given to the nurses and the hospital, the media attention focuses more favorably on forensics and allows the hospital to feel better about paying for the nurses to take these classes.

Lately, forensic nursing has been fraught with misunderstandings. Our scope of practice has been questioned more than it ever has in the twenty-five years since the sexual assault response teams, for example, were founded.

It is necessary that the law enforcement officers and courts be aware of what we are equipped to do so that they can use our skills to win their cases and clear our streets of criminals. In order to do this effectively, we need to be represented on all State Boards of Nursing by a forensic nurse, so that our evaluation of victims, our freedom to use the needed equipment and to find evidence is not hampered.

Our work as forensic nurses focuses on a variety of issues: domestic violence, sexual assault, homicide, death investigations, child abuse, workman's comp, vehicular injuries, elder abuse and neglect . . . and more.

This book is also for you, the public. Should you or someone you know suffer sexual assault, death, or other trauma, we want you to be aware of what the forensic nurse can do to ease your suffering and work toward getting justice. Forensic nurses work hard, but the hardest part is seeing the victims failed by the system. Join us, help us in defeating the violence. Let us make this a society we can be proud of. This book is written not only for other nurses who might want to pursue forensics as their careers, not only for the doctors and other medical professionals who need to understand who we are and what we do and the advantage to be gained by working together. This book is also written for the public, to whom we offer our forensic skills to better meet their needs.

As Kathy Bell, an IAFN past president, stated,

nurses reach out to the police and the law so that we can function as a team; educate others in the medical profession on what a medico-legal case is and how we can work on it together; and do more research into understanding violence and solving problems for crime victims. Like the police, we need to study the victims and their histories, to understand ways and reasons they are chosen as victims. We need to study domestic violence and its effect not only on the victims, but the children as well. We need to understand grief and the way it relates to death investigations and what we, as nurses, can do to help the survivors through the night.

We can dive into the police pool and they, in turn, can swim with us, so that all the victims dragged from the waters will be resuscitated by both.

Many of my friends and colleagues in forensic nursing have contributed cases to this book. While the facts are true, because of legal and ethical considerations, names, locations, and minor details have been changed, and it might read like fiction, but it's not. The most important facts are there. The passion with which these nurses work has not and never will change.

To further the efforts of forensic nursing, a portion of the proceeds from this book will be given to the IAFN for research and scholarship.

Trauma Nurse

The forensic nurse is usually to be found in the emergency room, but that is not the only part of the hospital where forensic skills may be needed. In fact, demands on the expertise of a forensic nurse could be useful in almost any area of nursing. This unique species of nurse can be found in ICUs, operating rooms, burn units, air transports, emergency medical units, disaster medical services, and more. And then there are the subspecies: nurse-attorneys and nurse–legal consultants who frequent law offices, insurance companies, precincts, the province of the district attorney or child welfare and workmen's compensation agencies—the list is a long one.

First, however, let's go to the ER, the place where many forensic nurses gain their experience. Traffic and pedestrian accidents probably constitute the majority of cases that come into the ER. The nurse who is trained to be aware of physical evidence beyond the strictly medical can often gather from that where and how the accident took place. Noticing and remembering exactly what the victim looked like when he or she arrived in the emergency room can be a critical point of evidence, and needs to be fully documented.

Beyond that first step, any attempt to reconstruct the events will, again, include the observations of the nurse, who is the first to see the patient and talk to the family members or to any witnesses there may be. She is usually also the first to handle the patient's clothing and other effects, and deal with the specimens that are to go to the lab.

Barbara, a member of the Emergency Nurses Association (ENA), was surprised at how many ER nurses knew nothing at all about forensic nursing. "You can't take it in nursing school, and there is no book on Forensics 101 for nurses. Unless you seek out the information at places like IAFN, or specific classes, you don't learn about protecting chain of custody." It was from various classes that Barbara learned the trick of getting paint chips out of an open wound with Post-it notes.

"The glue is not really that sticky, and you can preserve it in a folded paper, wrapped so that they won't fly around." She learned that the injury will sometimes contain the impression of the license plate. Measurements can tell her where the bumper of the car was when it hit the victim and where the victim was in relation.

In the ER, life-saving procedures for victims of violence are the same whether the violence is accidental, self-inflicted, or the result of an assault. How you deal with other than strictly medical observations—and such important things beyond the area of medicine as the victim's clothing—can make the difference between removing a criminal from the streets and leaving him (or her) free to attack again.

Sari was found lying in the street and brought to the ER, unconscious.

Because she had no identification on her, it took a while before people in the ER could find out who she was.

They stabilized the victim and made arrangements for her to be admitted to ICU. The nurse began folding up the clothes to move with the patient. (Unfamiliar with forensics, she didn't know that clothes needed to be packaged separately, especially in a case of unidentified trauma.) Sari's leather coat, which had been taken off as they tried to revive her, had been hung over a chair.

"Wait a minute," the nurse said. "Look at this." She pointed at the impression of a license plate, its mirror image stamped in the coat. "It looks like she was hit by a car. And at the height of the mark, I would guess it was a truck."

The investigator was ecstatic.

Luckily the coat had not been thrown into the corner or wadded up, or the impression might have disappeared forever. It helped to arrest the suspect.

In a similar case, a young girl injured in a hit-and-run accident was brought into the hospital. As she was being transferred from the ambulance stretcher onto the gurney, the nurse noticed what appeared to be flecks of paint on the stretcher.

With the help of the police, she carefully collected the flecks and put them into a paper bag. There were no witnesses to the accident, and the young girl died without ever regaining consciousness.

The flecks of paint were identified by the crime lab as having come from a specific make of car. When later identified, the car was matched with the paint chips. The loose chips fit perfectly into the nick on the fender of the suspected vehicle.

The nurse's alertness to the possible importance of this tiny piece of evidence helped to find and identify the car's driver. She hadn't been able to save the child's life but she assisted significantly in getting a dangerous driver off the streets.

The nurse's attention to detail accounted for her noticing the evidence and realizing its possible importance. She prevented any physical change of the evidence by careful packaging, and she maintained the chain of custody by handing the paper bag directly to the officer. She also avoided having to spend hours in court, since the police officer who had assisted her with collecting the material was able to testify to the details.

Gunshot wounds are another reason many people find themselves in the ERs of large metropolitan hospitals. "Very few residents or nurses are taught what to look for in an exit or entrance wound. They all want to pretend to be Quincy and give an opinion, but 90 percent of the time they are wrong. They will also use terms like 'cut' rather than 'laceration,' or visa versa, because they are trained to see surgical cuts and wounds, not violence.

"Most residents spend at best three months in the ER. Unless they're at a teaching hospital in a big city, they don't see nearly enough to train them in trauma. I was trained in a special course to identify entrance and exit wounds, and I still get it wrong sometimes," one nurse said. "I would never go up on the stand and testify positively, beyond any doubt, unless I was really that sure. Even then, I would hedge my bets. The human body does all sorts of tricks, and there are too many variables in wounds to always be 100 percent certain.

"In a ballistic case, or a homicide, we take the bullet and label it, sign it, and seal it. Then we hand it over to the police. It's important to know where that bullet came from, when we took it out, what the wound looked like, what the victim said, if anything. All this goes in the chart along with a reference to the bullet being given to detective so-and-so."

Hurried and concerned with life-saving procedures, a doctor might handle a bullet hole carelessly, not realizing the importance of keeping it untouched until it has been examined by the pathologist. In an effort to avoid doing more damage than necessary to a seriously injured man, a doctor has been known to forgo making a hole for a breathing tube; instead, he'd stick the tube through the hole the bullet had made. By draining the excess fluid, he'd prolong the victim's life, but in doing so he'd destroy the path of the bullet, making it harder to determine the angle at which the victim had been shot and hampering the reconstruction of the crime scene.

Items taken off a gunshot victim are also important for a number of reasons.

Alan, a nurse in the ER, was present when Mark, who had been shot in the head by an armed robber, was brought into the hospital. Mark was the third grocer to have been robbed that month. While the police suspected that all three crimes were perpetrated by the same gunman, they had no leads as to who the criminal might be.

Hoping that this victim might be able to provide some clues, a police officer accompanied the man into the hospital. He waited patiently in the lobby while Alan took over. Peeling back the temporary four-by-four bandages from the man's head, the nurse threw them into the trash bucket. He didn't notice the small metallic ringing sound as the gauze hit the garbage can.

When the patient was taken into the X-ray room, the officer asked Alan if anything had been discovered outside of the man's injuries when he examined the man.

"No, I don't think so . . ." He paused. "Wait a moment. I did hear something." He went to the trash. "When I was throwing away the dressings . . ." With his gloves still on, Alan looked through the trash can and found a spent bullet.

It was Alan's belated remembrance that led the police to the identification of the gunman and his arrest.

When the case came to court, however, the defense counsel had triumphantly made the point that the bullet was not discovered until the trash was checked.

"Why was it thrown away?" he asked.

"Because I was busy trying to staunch the bleeding and change the dressing, I didn't realize there was anything in with the bandages."

"When was the last time the trash can was emptied?"

"We empty if after every case, usually. I know it was clean when I put the four-by-fours in it."

"How many other gunshot wounds did you treat that day?"

"This was the first one."

"How do you know someone didn't put the bullet in the can while you were gone?"

"Of course that is always possible, but I didn't leave the room. When there is evidence, such as we had with this victim, I don't leave the room."

"You didn't leave the room?"

"Not until I turned the evidence over to the detective and it was then, when he came into the room, that we discovered the bullet in the trash."

The information about the bullet could not be tied beyond reasonable doubt to the gunman, because the bullet was not observed on the victim's body, but fortunately, a lineup identification led to his arrest and conviction.

♦ ♦ ♦

It's easy to mix up cuts and lacerations unless you are aware of the differences. A lot of nurses still do it, or they call them "gashes." But there are some very easy pointers to tell them apart.

Think of a watermelon. When you cut it with a knife, the edges are smooth, even, and if you had to close it again, you would see that the lines fit neatly together. If, on the other hand, you took a hammer and smashed the watermelon, it would fall apart in a million pieces. Some edges might be smooth, but most would be jagged and uneven. It would create a lot of problems if you tried putting that puzzle back together. Looking closely at the separation (before it totally falls apart), you'll find a bridging between the two main pieces. The bridging can be very tiny and hard to see unless you look closely, especially in a small wound. These are lacerations.

When a person, or a thing, is hit by a blunt object, say a baseball bat (or even a penis, as the cervix during rape), the force shatters or tears the object, depending on what the object is. Skin, being elastic to a degree, will bounce, stretch, and tear. Bone, on the other hand, will most likely break or shatter. This is a blunt-force trauma.

This may seem like trivia, but knowing these distinctions is very important when nurses and doctors chart wounds that are or might become part of legal cases.

After all, if I note on a chart that the patient had a

cut on his brow, that would imply it was made by a knife. The defendant does not have a knife. Therefore, the legal system assumes that the defendant is innocent. In fact, the victim's skin was broken when he was hit with a statue, which caused a laceration. Had the nurse written "laceration," the chances of the defendant's being found guilty might have increased.

Understanding patterns and patterned injury is crucial for nurses working in the emergency room. This knowledge, applied at the right moment, can save police work and lives.

Janet was working the ER the night that Edgar was brought in as a patient. Edgar was well known to the ER staff; he was a homeless man who made a habit of coming in with some complaint that the staff knew was simply an attempt to get a hot meal or just some company. If the ER wasn't busy that night, no one really minded.

That night, though, he didn't walk in; he was brought in by ambulance. The man was saturated with what was obviously gasoline and was mumbling incoherently.

"What happened, Edgar?"

He couldn't tell them. To their knowledge, Edgar did not use drugs. They could only assume that someone had tried to torch him and was interrupted just in time.

His blood alcohol was negative. Drug tests also proved negative.

"His oxygen level is low," the lab tech who was testing the gas levels in his blood said. That explained his disorientation, but how did that happen? Insufficient oxygen in the brain cells is enough to disrupt anyone's thinking. Perhaps the gasoline fumes had been the cause. There were enough chemical burns on his skin to indicate that the petroleum had been on his skin for several hours.

Examination showed that the burns and the saturation on Edgar's clothing were on the front of his torso, with only minimal amounts on his arms or shoulders. Inside his pockets, a cigarette lighter was found, but no matches, which was odd; no one had ever seen Edgar smoke.

This was the key to the puzzle. (This hypothesis was later confirmed when he regained consciousness and could speak to the ER staff.) The particular distribution of burns and gasoline indicated a suicide attempt. The ER staff concluded that poor Edgar had doused himself with gasoline and tried to set himself on fire, only partially succeeding. Overcome by the fumes, he had passed out and couldn't complete his effort.

Had they not come to this realization, the police would have been on a wild-goose chase, looking for the creep who tried to kill a homeless man, not knowing that the "creep" was Edgar himself.

Edgar was transferred to the psychiatric ward, where they helped him find a bed in a halfway house and get into a job-training program.

Neil was a young, healthy-looking man. He arrived by ambulance on a rainy afternoon after a neighbor discovered him lying unconscious on the ground in his yard. By the time the paramedics arrived, he was in full cardiac arrest. The medics managed to resuscitate him, but, despite their efforts, he kept returning to potentially lethal rhythms.

His wife told the ER staff that, to her knowledge, he had no history of medical problems or allergies.

During a lull in the effort of getting him stable, the medics managed to strip off his wet clothing and discovered two small burn marks on the inner part of his left ankle and on his left shoulder. They recognized the pattern. It was a lightning strike. The sheer amount of electrical energy that had passed through his body explained the dysfunctional activity of his heart.

The diagnosis came just in time. He went into another cardiac arrest as they were setting up the pacemaker and defibrillator that would put him on the road to recovery.

Part of police protocol in taking alleged perpetrators to jail is to take them to the emergency room and have them medically cleared. If the exam, or the perpetrators' accounts of their medical history have anything questionable whatsoever in it, they would be seen by a doctor.

One busy night a man was brought to the ER in handcuffs. He was accused of shooting and fatally wounding his girlfriend. The weapon had not been recovered.

Overwhelmed by cases that night, the ER doctor had only done a cursory interview and examination, but the nurse felt that something about this man did not seem right. He appeared to have an intermittent gait problem . . . that is, he walked strangely. He seemed very anxious to leave for the jail, and his demeanor was a bit too cooperative, considering the situation.

"Doctor, could you reexamine this suspect?" the nurse asked.

The doctor waved his hand toward the crowded waiting room.

The nurse nodded. She completely understood, and yet she didn't feel comfortable releasing Michael to the waiting officer.

Returning to the prisoner, she said, "You seem to be having trouble walking. Are you in pain?"

He gave her what he must have thought was the I'll-charm-the-pants-off-her smile.

She smiled back.

"I think before we send you on your way, we'd better do one more exam," she said. "I would hate to have the officer bring you all the way back here with some medical problem that we could easily have found."

With the doctor's permission, the nurse signed the order for an X-ray and a lower gastrointestinal scan.

The X-ray was all she needed.

Michael had concealed the murder weapon, still loaded, in his rectum. Who knows what other agenda he had planned for that night at the police station?

The officers were glad the nurse had noticed that something was not right and persisted in further examining the suspect before she released him to them.

◆ ◆ ◆

Jenny was a six-year-old who had been critically injured in a hit-and-run accident. The car had swerved into the yard where she was playing, and then sped away. Mom, who had been in the yard, too, had turned away from the girl for what had been the crucial second and could not identify the car other than with a vague description of its color.

As the ER staff instituted life-saving measures, they noticed a patterned injury on the child's back. Normally children tend to turn toward an oncoming vehicle and adults turn away. In all likelihood, Jenny never knew what hit her, but the pattern resembled the grillwork of a car.

Someone who has not witnessed this finds it hard to believe that the pattern can be so clear, but on many things, especially when enough force is used, the outlines give professional observers a fairly good picture. The crime lab was able to use the "picture" of the grillwork to ascertain the make of the car. Paint fragments found on the child's clothing (which had been properly collected) were matched to the make. Armed with this information, investigators found the car itself in a few days. There were traces of blood and fabric still in the grill.

The vehicle, it turned out, belonged to a friend of Jenny's mother. Jenny's father, her ex-boyfriend, had borrowed the car as well as the money for a bottle of liquid courage. He had drunk the whole bottle before deciding to pay Mom a visit.

He never knew he had struck his daughter.

Jenny recovered from her critical injuries but spent several months in intensive care before being released to rehab.

There is a craft to interviewing a patient, whether it is a victim or a suspect. The nurse quickly learns that leading questions can distract an interviewee and cause future problems. It is important that the person doing the interview avoid these at all costs.

Marta, a thirteen-year-old, had an IQ just above retarded but that didn't prevent her father, now divorced from the mother, for wanting the visitation rights for "his girl." After a five-day visit with him, the girl and her mother came into the emergency room because Marta was complaining that her "pee-pee was sore from Daddy."

The pediatrician on call did not hide his distaste for a potential sexual assault case and admitted that he had only minimal knowledge of the correct way to collect and preserve evidence. Nevertheless, he refused to let the SANE on call that night do the exam.

"It's probably nothing anyway," he told the mother and the nurse.

Once inside, listening to the doctor talking to the patient, the SANE cringed. The pediatrician's questions were:

"Is your private place sore because Daddy wiped you too hard?"

"Does it itch down there?"

"Do you scratch it a lot?"

His examination below the patient's waist was cursory. Finding a bit of tissue on her labia, he explained to the mother, "See, your daughter is merely wiping herself too hard."

Carolyn, the SANE, was horrified at the clumsiness of the exam, but there was nothing she could do in front of the doctor. In private, however, she asked the mother to come back the next night with her daughter and bring with her some of the clothes that the girl had worn during her five days with her father.

Reporting off to Jennifer, the SANE who would be on call the next night, Carolyn voiced her suspicions and told Jennifer what instructions she had given the mother. Carolyn had already checked the schedule. The pediatrician on call for the next night was one of the few ones at the hospital who had supported the SANE program.

The next night the mother and daughter came back, Mom carrying six bags of clothes, each holding a separate item. The mother had asked the girl to pick out the clothes she had worn the most and what she had worn when she told Daddy that her "pee-pee hurt."

Jennifer examined the girl and found vaginal redness and some swelling, which she documented with photos and recorded descriptions. The most telling part of all, however, was the result of the crime lab's test for semen. Although the majority of the clothes showed negative, two pieces of clothing had spots of the substance and one had a large spill of the substance down the front.

The father confessed and is still doing time.

The doctor who refused to do a proper exam was called into court as a witness for the defense, only to be made a fool of when he had to admit that he had not done a real exam at all.

The nurse wanting to photograph a patient's injuries or tell-tale features of the body must get the patient's signature on a consent form first. Sometimes this is difficult to do, but the importance of photographs as evidence can't be overlooked. This raises some questions. Can we take photos of a patient who is unconscious? The photographs are crucial if the incident develops into a major case. If we can get a family member to sign the consent, we go with that. Otherwise, we often go ahead with the camera shots, giving the results to the police as part of the case. If there is an objection, we'll deal with that later.

"I had to learn everything from the ground up. I was making mistakes and no one had educated me on how to gather evidence," a nurse says. "One of the first big cases I had was a death. It wasn't a homicide, but it did introduce me to the world of forensic nursing.

"A big-dig tunnel worker was hit when a cement block fell on his head. He was killed instantly. Eventually there were several deaths on that dig—this man's was one of the first.

"The police, the construction company's lawyer,

everyone wanted the victim's clothes, his lab data, and tox screens. This wasn't a murder investigation of any sort, and so I didn't even realize that something like this was forensic. Obviously it was, since the dig was investigated to see if the company could be blamed for inadequate safety for the workers. That made me aware that even if the police aren't really involved in an episode, it still could be a medical-legal case. I wanted to make sure that I did everything right for the family and not have it come back to haunt me."

Six police officers had been lost that year already. When the man suspected of the two most recent homicides was brought into the emergency room, the staff knew their observations would be crucial for the prosecution at the trial that would follow.

Two forensic nurses were assigned to this case to make sure that nothing was missed.

Observations they made of each suspect included eye contact, demeanor, signs of abuse or injury, tone of voice, affect, general appearance, including the condition of his clothing, and debris on the clothing and shoes.

They also checked for abrasions, contusions, gunpowder burns to the hands, and debris under the nails. All of these things were meticulously documented in the event that a suspect later made a claim of police brutality or an insanity plea.

As it turned out, one of the suspects did both. The ER staff were able to point to the photos that they had taken of his injuries as such, and surmised how they could have most probably been made in his effort to run from the police rather than as the result of police abuse. The debris under his nails, the crime lab determined, was from scaling a wall during his escape.

To counter his insanity plea, they pointed out that someone wearing clothes in as good a condition, and as clean and pressed as his were, did not indicate any mental disorder—other than his misconception that he had a right to shoot up stores and the police who tried to stop him.

Use of more than one forensic nurse was justified when it turned out that each of them found details that her partner had not noticed. Just because a forensic nurse is trained doesn't mean she will catch all the subtle clues that exist.

Patrick was a middle-aged man who was brought in as the victim of an assault. He had multiple stab wounds to his chest. Although he had told his wife that he had been attacked, the fifteen cuts on his body were in what immediately seemed a suspicious pattern. They matched the reach of his dominant hand plus the length of a sharp object, and were far from deep; they were superficial wounds. It was clear to the forensic nurse that the wounds were self-inflicted, the result of either a genuine suicide effort or a false one. When the ER staff saw the old horizontal scars on each wrist, they knew their "educated guess" was confirmed.

Patrick seemed more concerned that his wife remain in the waiting room and not be given the findings about his condition than he was with his survival. It was obvious that he wanted her to feel sorry for him. But the medics' observations uncovered the truth and prevented the police from trying to find and arrest an innocent person.

Crimes against other humans will force the nurse to decide which obligations are due the patient and which the law. When the patient is in the hospital setting, we are urged to preserve his or her privacy, and so the nurse may have to decide to collect or release evidence. The delay can cause the physical evidence to be useless or make the collection impossible.

The decision of a victim who refuses photographs has, by law, to be obeyed. In such a case, the nurse or doctor may be subpoenaed to testify that the request was made and the victim refused it. However, courts have ruled that once the victim is moved from the ER, any trace evidence that remains on the sheet (e.g., hair fibers, blood) can be taken by the police, since privacy is not deemed violated by this. In such cases, it is even more important that the nurse's charting accurately reflect the patient's condition, appearance, and attitude. (With unconscious patients, DAs have ruled, in more than one instance, that evidence can be gathered. In a case where gastric lavage had to be done to save the patient's life, for example, the DA ordered the stomach's contents to be saved as evidence. Even if the DA had not ordered this, the nurse should have done so; it could have been important evidence in the future.)

Sometimes the choice is a hard one. In one case, where it appeared that the unconscious patient had been the victim of an assault or a similar criminal act, the nurse, protecting the evidence, turned the woman's clothing over to the police. When the woman regained consciousness, she claimed that her rights had been violated, because she didn't plan to press charges.

A case arose when a driver, whose actions indicated alcohol intake, was brought into the ER. After an accident, the police asked that his blood level be drawn, but he refused to cooperate. Because determining his blood alcohol level was not a medical necessity, the nurse didn't want to do it against his wishes without a direct order from the district attorney. Maybe it was her nurse's instinct, because while she was talking to him, she noticed something. Although the room was fairly cool, he was sweating and showing other symptoms of low blood sugar (hypoglycemia). This could be an indication of diabetes rather than of intoxication. The patient was so grateful that diabetes was discovered and he could go into treatment before any real damage had been done, he did not even sue the officer for false arrest.

The nurse needs to know how to question a patient in order to get accurate information.

Jen was working the night that Gerald S., a worker at a local factory, was admitted to the trauma center after a car accident. Reportedly, he had lost control of the car, which had left the road and hit a concrete divider head-on. Gerald had not been wearing his seat belt.

He had a possible pelvic fracture and injury to his left lung and heart. His injuries were consistent with sudden stopping of the car while the body continues to fly through the air.

"Leave me alone," Gerald demanded as Jen tried to start the IV.

"Mr. S., we have to give you this medication; your heart is beating erratically."

"I don't care. I don't want anything. Just leave me alone."

Gerald had no evidence of trauma to his head, which might have caused his combative attitude. Testing his B.A. (blood alcohol) at 0.07 showed the nurse a cause for his unreasonableness.

The detective entered to report that at the site of the crash there were no skid marks, which would have indicated that the driver tried to stop suddenly. "He must have fallen asleep at the wheel."

"Perhaps," the nurse said. "That could be one possibility for the absence of skid marks. He could have had a heart attack, too, but so far the reports don't show that."

Gerald's wife was very adamant when told he hadn't been wearing a seat belt. "That can't be. He's always insisting that everyone buckle up. I can't believe he would have driven without it . . . unless . . ." Her voice suddenly cracked. Tears came to her eyes. "It must have been my fault. We argued early today. He's under such stress at work with this new job and all. I should have been more understanding. But you know," she added, "other than during our argument this morning, he was in a pretty good mood."

Jen knew that deeply depressed patients often don't have the energy to carry out their suicidal plans but, as the depression lifts, they have more ability to act, even though the sense of helplessness still remains.

"Well, his physical injuries don't seem to be critical, but I think the doctor is going to transfer him upstairs for some observation," she said. "I'll check to find out when you can talk with him." Since Jen suspected a suicide attempt, she knew that it was not a good idea to leave the patient alone. One failed attempt did not mean the patient wanted to live. In fact, victims who have succeeded at suicide often have a history of failed attempts.

Just before transferring Gerald to the trauma care unit for treatment of his physical injuries, Jen confronted him with the facts and her observations about the crash. Her questions were kindly, but they left little room for misunderstanding.

"Gerald, are you so unhappy with your life right now that you tried to hurt yourself?"

"So what if I did? Obviously I failed. I'm still alive."

"Would you like to talk with someone about your feelings?"

He glared at her. "No." Suicide patients will seldom volunteer the information that they have tried to kill themselves, but they will usually not deny it.

Two days later the psychiatric nurse came up to speak with him. It was the wrong moment. His wife was with him.

Gerald denied that he had any suicidal intent. "I would never do such a thing," he said.

"He was just distracted because of our argument," the wife said, taking the blame for everything.

"Have you had other accidents recently?" the psychiatric nurse asked.

"Yes, he's been rather accident-prone lately. He . . ." the wife started to answer until a look from her husband silenced her.

It appeared pretty clear to the nurse that Gerald had made at least one failed suicide attempt before his accident.

As it turned out, Jen, having been trained as a forensic nurse, saved Gerald's clothes and shoes as evidence. She was able to show that the sole of Gerald's right shoe had the imprint of the gas pedal and not the brake, as it might have if he truly had tried to stop.

A review of the patient's recent ER visits in the past year came up with two additional similar events. With the evidence in her hand, Jen was able to show Gerald's doctor that Gerald was suicidal.

Once he was physically stable, Gerald was taken to the psychiatric ward on a seventy-two-hour evaluation hold to determine whether he was at risk to himself or to others. Had Jen not been aware of the signs and the evidence, Gerald might have made another attempt.

The emergency room often deals with burn victims. Gary, who works with the National Forensic Burn Unit (NFB), is a former police officer. "In the police academy, we were taught to go to the M.D. 'What do you think?' we would ask. We would then build the case based on what the doctor alleged. No one thought that some injuries could be purely accidental, but sometimes they were. Now, with the NFB, we take the forensic water temperature, ask about the recovery cycle of the water heater, and take a social history of those involved. A number of people who have been wrongly accused of child abuse have had retrials because of us."

As expert witnesses both for the defense and prosecution, the forensic nurses of NFB turn away more cases than they accept now, but it wasn't always this way. As nurses, even with advanced training, they've had to do quite a bit of convincing to get approved as experts. "One of our nurses got a Ph.D. in pharmacology so we could address her as doctor. She was one of the first ones to break the ice."

Most of the nurses at the NFB also do arson cases. When someone dies in a fire, they can tell by the burn if the victim was dead or alive at the time of the burn. Dead tissue will burn faster and deeper, because there is no vascular support from the blood supply.

"There are all sorts of variations that will affect how a burn will look," Gary says. "When six-year-old Patrick was brought into the ER with a deep burn on his hand and a clear line around his wrist, the staff thought of child abuse and immediately accused the mother. But what had happened was that Patrick had put his hand into the frying pan. Hot oil or grease, being thicker and more viscous, will adhere to the skin.

The burn goes deeper because the temperature can't dissipate as quickly as it would if it had just been hot water on the skin. Patrick's burns had been the result of an accident.

"Since the NFB is centered in New Jersey, almost every child who comes to our office for an opinion comes through the Department of Protective Services. We have an agreement with DAs and prosecutors throughout the United States to handle child-protective civil and criminal cases. The nurses here now train law enforcement and social workers, as well as other members of the judiciary system who investigate or render opinions in burn cases.

"Even the advanced practice nurse—the NP, or nurse practitioner—in the community hospital does not have the experience with burns that we do."

Specialists in forensic burns get not only education in burn treatment—hydrotherapy, dressing burns, and use of topical ointments. They are also taught how to test the water temperature, how to measure the height and fixture of the burn, the thermal dissipation of the burn, the types of pipes in the house and heating system. "You can tell if a child was restrained and how long they were in contact with the thermal source, if you know what to test." Everything comes into play, including any medication that the burn victim was using. Not even medical experts are aware of some of these factors.

"One young girl was cautioned to stay out of the sun, since the antidepressant that she was taking could make it easy for her to burn. In addition, a burn she received when she slipped in a tub of hot water was more severe than it would have been had she not been on the medication. Only a person trained in forensic burns would know this."

Sometimes the item that gives the patient a burn leaves a clear mark.

Fifteen-year-old Karin had been babysitting for her little brother, Eric. She really wanted to go out with her friends and had planned on sneaking away after he was asleep.

But instead of going to bed as he should have, Eric began to play with Karin's makeup and refused to stop. Enraged, Karin put her hot curling iron to his hand, burning him.

When he wouldn't stop crying, she thrust him into his crib.

Unable to stand the noise, she silenced him with a pillow over his face, and was relieved when, after a few minutes, he quieted.

Lucky for Eric, the phone rang.

It was one of Karin's friends, making sure that the girl was still going out with them that night.

Eric regained consciousness, crawled out of the crib, and hid until his sister left.

Ann, the forensic nurse who examined Eric in the emergency room when his mother brought him in later that night, quickly identified a curling iron as the cause of the burn, and took photos. "Sometimes the object doesn't photograph picture-perfect," Ann said, "but a comparison with the original object will almost always show you the truth."

How deep the burn is will often depend on how long it was exposed to the thermal heat source, and the forensic-trained nurse is equipped to judge the depth of the burn as the doctor is cleaning the burned tissue away from the wound. A wound beyond a certain depth would be an indication that it was caused by child abuse. Photos need to be taken before the cleaning process, known as the debridement, takes place, since the configuration of the burn changes once the doctor starts excising the dead tissue.

Those who work for the NFB are trained to differentiate burns at different stages, to collect evidence properly, and to take forensic photos.

"Sometimes what we are looking at is not a burn at all, although it might look like one," Ann says, relating the case of a patient who had an allergic condition. By taking samples of the skin, she was able to tell that this was not a true burn, and the mother was not accused of abuse.

"Just as with other trauma, saving any clothes the victim was in can make or break a case."

Carol Sue had fallen into a tub of very hot water and burned her hand. There was a clear line of demarcation on the child's wrist. Although child abuse was first considered, the actual happening was soon worked out: the baby had been wearing an outfit with a long sleeve, and elastic on the wrist did not let the hot water get through to injure the rest of her arm. What she was wearing when she fell into the tub was verified by the imprint of the garment seam and of its zipper on the child's body.

Thanks to the work of the National Forensic Burn Center, more and more nurses are being used today on arson investigation cases, and more people that would have been accused of abuse are freed.

Since it is often unclear whether a patient's condition is the result of an accident or of a crime, the nurse caring for the patient needs to be aware of several things:

Remember that the body is a crime scene. This is especially true when any violence involves what could be abuse of a child, an elderly person, or a domestic partner. If a court case ensues, or if the victim dies, the actual use of violence can be shown to have taken place by prompt charting and proper evidence.

Retain any evidence. This means carefully keeping *all* evidence properly until the police have cleared it completely. Never mind the pleas of relatives; they must wait until law enforcement is finished with it. This includes anything that comes in with the victim and any dressings or clothing that the victim has worn during the attack. It also includes the sheets or newspapers that the victim has stood upon and any debris found on the body or clothing. Often the simple things can help determine what has really happened. Holes and tears in a victim's clothing offer an important way to verify the story and reconstruct a crime scene. It's a clue if the dimensions of the hole in the clothing match the bullet that reportedly has been fired.

Prevent changes in the physical condition of evidence. Items should be handled as little as possible. Each item should be wrapped separately to avoid transferring of trace evidence from one item to another. For instance, if paint chips from the car that hit the victim were on the coat, but the coat got wrapped with the other clothes, it would be hard to tell where the paint chips had fallen from. It could be assumed, or made an issue of, by the defense, who would say that the paint chips might have been on the inner clothing, that the car had not hit the victim or had not been the one identified, or that the paint had come from someplace else. Clothes that are thrown into a pile can also contaminate the evidence in a case of rape or assault. Blood stains transferred from one garment to another can confuse investigators and jurors. A piece of pubic hair falling from the victim's underwear means something very different from one that's fallen from another piece of his or her clothing. It could ID the suspect, but if it has come from another part of the clothing, the defense could easily challenge that with another story to match the find.

Keep proper documentation. That includes photos and written notification of what photos were taken, especially if they were given to the police.

Maintain the chain of custody. Potential evidence can't be left unattended even for a moment. If it is, the evidence is invalidated. Have someone assist you or back you up if you have to leave the room.

Have all the procedures witnessed. Police officers are the best placed to assist or take care of this aspect. Properly done, it obviates the necessity of the nurse's court appearance.

Get names and addresses of everyone accompanying the victim. The simple process of making sure you have gotten names and addresses of all people who bring or accompany the victim to the hospital can aid the prosecuting attorney.

Many decisions that nurses have to make in the ER or just in their day-to-day routines are forensically oriented, even if the nurses aren't aware of that because they haven't been trained in forensics.

Every bodily fluid, every human cell that has been shed, and every smudge on skin or clothing carries a potential story in trace evidence in the city crime lab.

While physical evidence is sometimes the most valuable data in solving a crime, it is also the most easily lost. Blood stains, semen, or dirt disappear in the flick of a washcloth. Urine collected one hour after a crime varies greatly from that collected eight hours later. Forensics and the emergency room go hand in hand.

The Sexual Assault Nurse Examiner

Absence of evidence is not evidence of absence.
—Carl Sagan

The most common subspecies of the forensic nurse is the sexual assault nurse examiner (SANE).

A significant percentage of patients who come into the emergency room of a hospital are victims of sexual assault and/or rape.

The approach to sexual assault exams varies greatly, depending on where it takes place. Methods differ from city to city, state to state, and even hospital and/or SART locations. Although different cities and practice groups had various routines for examining victims of rape and other trauma, the SANE nurses were unanimous in believing that there was a better way than the present practice to help victims and survivors. Pioneering nurses began to organize.

This has resulted in the increase in the numbers of nurses who specialize in the forensics of these crimes—

the SANEs. Some newer programs have chosen to use the more generic term of sexual assault/forensic examiner (SAFE) or forensic nurse examiner (FNE). The SANE is not to be confused with the rape advocate. Almost all rape advocates are volunteers, and their primary duty is to comfort and support the victim emotionally. They are trained to take the side of the victim, a service that is enormously helpful to the victims of assault and rape. SANEs and nurse practitioners, however, have a different purpose. First, of course, they must be registered nurses. Along with their discovery of the patient's trauma, which must be called to the attention of the doctor, their job is to find the facts, to protect the evidence and learn what it shows.

Many SANEs may begin as emergency room nurses who don't want to go beyond strictly medical care of the victims of rape and assault, but after working awhile with this type of patient, they find themselves becoming advocates for them. They become willing to spend three to six hours in the sexual assault exam room, incurring the wrath of colleagues and doctors, being challenged by defense attorneys in a courtroom trial. How they work and how they help the police is the subject of this chapter.

I had been speaking to a group of high school students about aspects of rape and the necessity of a SANE-performed proper forensic exam, including the collection of evidence. A hand went up in the audience.

"What would you do if your son was accused of raping someone?"

"Well, if I had a son, here is what I would do: First I would want to know all the facts of the incident from both parties, not just his side. I would insist that both he and the woman have a full exam performed by a sexual assault nurse. I would want all the evidence to be collected. If possible, I would see to it that neither he nor the woman washed before being examined, and that they were still wearing the clothing they'd had on at the time of the episode, if possible, since clothing can be a source of trace evidence. Then I'd take photographs and test swabs of any area that she claimed was touched, and any other areas that are commonly touched, just in case she had forgotten one or more."

"What if your son said it wasn't rape? What if he said it was consensual? Wouldn't you believe him?"

I shook my head. "As much as I would like to believe him, everyone has a different perception of events. The man who sees a young woman scantily dressed on the street can tell himself that she is asking for it, that she wants it, and that she is leading him on. A man who has a fetish for young girls might say that their tight clothes are seducing him. It is his perception only.

"The fact is no one asks to be a victim of violence.

"I would have to believe the physical evidence. That is what almost always tells us whether the stories match what the participants have told. Evidence of a consensual sexual act will be different from evidence of rape."

"What kind of mother are you not to support your child?" someone else demanded.

"I couldn't support him automatically because, as I said, physical evidence doesn't lie. Every time we touch someone, trace evidence is transferred. Even if I touch the microphone, my fingerprints and tiny flecks of my saliva transfer. If what he says contradicts what she says, and I find evidence that proves her story is correct, I have to believe her.

"Certainly I would be very sad to find my son capable of rape, but I would also want him to get treatment and make sure that such a thing did not happen again."

"What if she was lying because she was angry at your son?" the other person insisted.

"The physical evidence would prove what happened. I would have to listen to that. It's true that many parents want to believe their children innocent of wrongdoing. But if the physical evidence shows us that something was possible, if there are injuries that would not have happened with consensual sex, than I would have no choice but to believe the facts. My son would be justly punished for what he had done and we would deal with the consequences."

I continued to stress how important it is that rape victims not change clothes or wash away the evidence afterward, no matter how dirty and unclean they might feel. The more evidence is there, the easier it is to get a conviction. Of course, in some cases no physical evidence can be recovered. But usually there is something in the telling of what happened that will give you clues.

In fact, more than 80 percent of victims who receive a proper SANE exam have a successful prosecution of the rapist. It's also true that there are cases of false arrest; what seems to be the proof is misinterpreted by the investigators, and it is soon shown that there is no reason to proceed any further. On the other hand, when the guilty party is faced with the facts, he will often confess to the rape immediately.

The International Association of Forensic Nurses (IAFN) has developed scope and standards of forensic nursing practice. These standards include, among other things, the definition of the SANE's practice area, what constitutes a forensic exam, and how we are supposed to evaluate and document (with photos and written reports) our findings. A copy of this report can be obtained for a nominal fee from the IAFN office in New Jersey. (Addresses are listed in the acknowledgments.)

All SANEs are registered nurses with advanced skills in the care of sexual assault patients. Some are graduates of two- or three-year nursing schools with an additional good deal of hands-on experience; some are nurses with bachelor degrees trained to think more theoretically. Some are even nurse practitioners or have doctorates in nursing. Regardless of their status on the nursing ladder, they all are trained in productive ways to interview patients and suspects and to regard the stories of both with cautious skepticism.

The forty-plus-hour class in sexual assault nursing includes information and training not only in taking a basic patient medical history and a physical exam, but also interview techniques, hands-on specula exams with emphasis on identifying wounds and patterned injuries, evidence collection, courtroom testimony, forensic photography, examining for domestic violence, child abuse, and proper documentation of the entire examination of the patient. It sometimes also includes a "ride-along" with the local police.

The SANE program operates on the belief that all victims have the right to immediate, compassionate, unbiased, and comprehensive medical-legal evaluation and treatment by skilled professionals who can anticipate their needs during this crisis. Victims of sexual assault get knowledgeable support as they wade through the criminal justice system, a journey that can sometimes be at least as hard on the victim as on the suspect or perpetrator. That is why the SANEs work with and stay with the victim throughout a trial and beyond.

The majority of the sexual assault victims are attacked by someone they know, which means that many of these cases are "date rapes" or are committed by some more or less "friendly" acquaintance. Most SANE nurses also have training in "victimology": They can help the police to find connections between active cases and thus get a better picture of an unknown rapist.

Malinda, an ER nurse in a large municipal hospital, felt deeply aggrieved by the way the all-too-frequent rape cases that came into her emergency room were handled. Often the necessary police follow-up was missing or done sketchily, evidence was contaminated or even not recognized and discarded. The patient would have been allowed to wash, which would obliterate many of the bodily signs of probable rape, and more possibilities of telltale evidence was being overlooked, not photographed, and so on. Malinda worried about this. She knew there must be a better way to take care of rape victims. Only she wasn't sure what it was.

Then she went to a lecture given by Virginia Lynch. The subject was forensic insight of trauma nursing. To Malinda, it was a revelation. What the rape patient needed was a sexual assault response team (SART).

"You'll never do it. You'll fall flat on your face," the rape advocate director told her. "Honey, don't you think I've tried? I've been trying for years to get somewhere with the police. Give up. I have. They just walk right past and ignore everything I've done. And I have more clout than you do in this town."

But Malinda, who as nurse practitioner was almost at the top of her professional career, would not take "no" for an answer.

Starting out in 1994 with guidance and support from Virginia Lynch and others in the budding forensic nursing organization, Malinda went forth like Joan of Arc, with her banner high. Now, almost ten years later, Malinda works out of two different hospital sites and is the owner of a private forensic nurse consulting company.

At the beginning, one of her biggest challenges came from the doctors. They didn't like the nurses taking over caring for rape patients, which they thought was their function, even though they had seldom done it and did not like doing it when they had to. "They ignored these victims and now they want us to ignore them." She fought back. "RNs should be doing the sexual assault cases . . . RNs who have been specifically trained to do these exams." She began training a core of people to work with her before she was even sure she would have a center to work from.

Slowly the police were starting to call Malinda for advice. Slowly both parties learned to respect each other's jobs.

The other problem these "rape nurses" had was getting paid for court time. For the most part, Malinda's nurses came to court not just as accessory witnesses, but also as expert witnesses. They would spend hours before the trial and then, later, in the courtroom, going over the case in question with the district attorney's staff members. Now, she will not take a contract from the local law enforcement unless they agree to pay for testimony time as well, and they pay, aware that she is valuable to them.

Even so, the nurses are still not paid what they are worth. Most of those who want to serve the public as nurse investigators have to take a cut in pay to do this. They can't afford to leave their other jobs, but they are dedicated to this special work. Compared to what a nurse practitioner gets at a hospital—$30–$40 per hour a usual rate in 2003—they have to accept as little as $8 an hour for participating as witnesses in a court case. (Many of them even simply start off as volunteers.) But this situation cannot remain static. "If we want quality people, we have to pay, or else the good ones will burn out," Malinda says. "Our court rate takes only 12–14 percent of the time away from our hospital job; most of our nurses document so thoroughly that often the perp pleads out before we get to court."

Out of 350 victims Malinda's nurses saw last year, 107 went through the court process and 97 completed trial with a 97 percent conviction rate. In the other rape cases, the accused rapists either confessed or pleaded to lesser charges, or the victim recanted her story or refused to press charges—or dropped out of sight.

Malinda urges her rape victims, "Don't be afraid to let the system work. Don't be afraid to tell someone. Don't be afraid to go through the process."

Marilyn, a twenty-two-year-old college student came to the emergency room late on a Saturday night. Her initial complaint was vaginal soreness and bleeding.

Lucky for her, Alexandra, a SANE, happened to be working the 11 p.m.–7 a.m. shift that night. After taking Marilyn's blood pressure and other vital signs, the nurse took her to the back room reserved for sexual assault exams.

In most, if not all states, nurses are mandated by law to report crime-related injuries to law enforcement. In addition, the policy of many SART programs is to call the rape advocate immediately; the client can decline the advocate's services after they meet.

Here Marilyn would be able to talk to the nurse in private, away from the prying ears of other patients and staff.

"Do you want to tell me when this soreness started?" Alexandra asked. She had a sealed rape–sexual assault evidence kit within reach, although she couldn't do anything without her patient admitting that she had been raped and consenting to a forensic evidence examination, but she wanted to be ready.

Marilyn shook her head. "My mind's a blank," she said. "I went to a party on Friday night with some of my friends and I . . . I don't remember what happened after that."

Alexandra nodded. "Did anyone give you anything to drink at the party? Or did you leave your drink alone for any length of time?"

"Just when I went to the bathroom," Marilyn said. "But my friends were at the table," she protested.

"Did they say anything about anyone coming near your drink?"

She shook her head. "I don't know. I didn't even think to ask."

"Marilyn, what do you think happened to you?" Alexandra asked. She saw no signs of cuts, bruises, or other physical injury, but that didn't mean nothing had happened.

The young woman shrugged. In a small voice, Marilyn said, "I think I was raped. I mean I . . ." Her voice trembled. "There was this guy staring at me all night at the party. I don't remember what he looked like."

Alexandra kept her voice calm. She could see the victim was becoming agitated. "Would you like to make a report to the police?" she asked quietly.

Marilyn shrugged. "I don't know. I mean, who will believe me? I don't have any proof. I—" There was a moment of hesitation. She obviously did not quite trust the nurse.

Alexandra sat down opposite the troubled young woman. "I can't say for sure, Marilyn, until I examine you, but it is quite possible you were raped. You could have been given one of those drugs that make you forget what happened."

"There are drugs that can do that?"

Alexandra nodded. "If you would like me to call the police, I can do so," she said. "I can also call the rape crisis line and have an advocate here with you while I, someone from the police, and the doctor talk to you."

"I . . . I don't know." Marilyn hesitated. "I'm still not really sure anything happened." She shrugged again, her voice barely audible. "Maybe I just imagined it all. Maybe I'm getting my period or something?" she suggested hopefully.

"And maybe something really did happen. You know, if it did, you could be saving a lot of other women trouble. And you would help the police build a case, perhaps get this person off the streets."

There were tears in Marilyn's eyes now. "But I didn't even see what he looked like. I don't have any idea who he is. I don't remember anything. I don't even know if anything really happened." She pushed herself off the gurney. "Maybe I should just go home and stop being a problem."

Alexandra put her hand gently on Marilyn's shoulder. "I tell you what. Why don't you let me do the exam? If I find something, if there is something that can possibly help the police find out who the man is . . . I can call them. Even if we don't find definite proof, you still might feel better if you make a report. And it would allow us to check for any sexually transmitted disease. Also, our program includes an offer of the morning-after pill, if you'd like to make sure no pregnancy results from your experience."

"Yeah, maybe," Marilyn sighed.

"Have you showered since the incident?"

The young woman shook her head. "When I got home I was so groggy that I fell right back to sleep. It was my roommate who insisted I go. She drove me over when I woke up."

"Where are the clothes you were wearing the night you went to the party?"

Marilyn indicated that she wore them still. "I was too shocked, too upset to do anything."

"Okay. I understand how you are feeling. It's good that you did not shower, because that would have washed away evidence. I'm also glad that you are wearing the same clothes, since we might find something in or on your clothing that could corroborate your story." Alexandra took out her Polaroid camera for instant pictures, and the 35-mm Nikon with the macro lens, which she used for photo documentation of bruises and injuries.

On the colposcope, which she would use later, Alexandra had a third camera, another 35-mm mounted for taking magnified photos of any injuries. This, too, could later be blown up and used in court.

Originally the colposcope had been used only for detecting vulval cancer. In recent years, doctors had started using it to also document child abuse. But with the start of the SANE program, and the research done by Dr. Laura Slaughter, it had become a standard of practice for identifying genital trauma associated with adult rape and sexual assault.

As a result of the colposcopic photos, victims with injuries invisible to the naked eye are now able to bring proof into court and see justice done. It was true that some saw the instrument as yet another blow to a patient's privacy, but careful preparation by the nurse and the rape advocate had minimized the predicted doom and gloom.

Despite the research, there were still facilities (she knew of one in a southern state) that did not have, did not use, or did not believe in the colposcope's ability. Moreover, one site went so far as to say that they would not even consider performing a rape exam on someone who was intoxicated with alcohol or drugs. Though the nurses there were trained as SANEs, they would have to base their judgments on such not-very-reliable factors as the way the victim dressed, the places she went, the time she went someplace, or whether she allowed herself to be picked up as a hitchhiker.

Alexandra was shocked when a nurse from that area said that she was disappointed in women victims for making themselves targets. To Alexandra's thinking, no one was asking to be a victim of violence, not even if they went into the street naked.

Alexandra hoped that Marilyn would file a report with the police. Her reason was partly selfish. Since their sexual response assault team was hospital-based, their funding was not independent. If no report was filed, in this jurisdiction, the hospital would not be paid for the three to six hours it would take to perform a complete forensic evidentiary exam. Neither did they get their supplies reimbursed, and Alexandra would not receive her SANE stipend for her time and her report.

But even if, by the end of the exam, Marilyn continued to hesitate, Alexandra would still need to fill the Department of Justice seven-page forms, including the sexual assault exam report with the chain of custody paperwork; the evidentiary exam consent, which also included a consent to release evidence to and communicate with law enforcement; pregnancy prevention consent; laboratory forms, including a specimen chain of custody; and follow-up materials.

It was not unheard of for a victim to return in a few days, maybe even in a few months and say she changed her mind. The completed rape kit would be kept up to thirty days.

However, if Alexandra did not take the specimens correctly now, there would be nothing to pursue . . . and maybe another girl or woman would find herself in Marilyn's situation, but worse.

Fear, Alexandra had learned, could motivate some of these victims to do just what the offender asks of them, which is often a reason that evidence of a struggle is not found.

Even if the victim felt she could not report the crime, just being at the ER with a skilled SANE would speed her recovery and prevent any secondary injury or illness. She had the right to the same medical care as someone who made a report.

After taking a preliminary medical history and a history of the events as the patient recalled there, Alexandra explained to Marilyn that she would be doing a brief physical exam.

Only minor injuries and those that she could document as items of possible forensic evidence would be of concern. "If I think there is anything the doctor should know, I will have him come in and see you before you are signed out. If there is any injury that I cannot deal with simply, I will call the doctor. If medications are needed, perhaps to prevent conception, he will prescribe them."

Had Marilyn come into the ER with blood loss, unconscious, or with numerous physical injuries, her care would be the responsibility of the emergency room doctors, and Alexandra could only hope that they would be careful to save clothing and whatever evidence they found. The nurse would only be able to do the sexual assault exam after the victim had been stabilized.

She was glad this was not the case tonight, since the doctor on call had not shown much support to the SANE program. He had a phobia of courts and therefore avoided becoming involved with anything that might bring him into contact with the justice system.

Alexandra took her first photos while the patient sat, and then had the young woman stand on two sheets spread out on the floor. This was to collect any evidence that might fall from her clothes as she disrobed and put on the hospital gown for the exam. Then pictures were taken as Marilyn stood.

So far, no injuries were visible to Alexandra's naked eye. But that didn't mean nothing had happened. And it didn't mean nothing existed. Carl Sagan had said, "Absence of evidence is not evidence of absence." Bruises sometimes took hours or days to develop.

As a skilled SANE, Alexandra had been trained to assess injury, objectively document the health history to determine the risk of medical and psychological problems, objectively document the history of the crime, screen for sexually transmitted diseases, collect and preserve forensic data, and, by making the proper referrals, help the patient/victim regain control of her life.

As Marilyn undressed, Alexandra put each item of clothing into a separate paper bag. Items that were damp from sweat, blood, or any other substance would be air-dried before being wrapped and stored. The paper bags kept evidence from degrading too rapidly. Plastic often erodes the evidence and destroys it.

Until such time as she had sealed the bags with evidence tape, dated them, labeled, signed with her name and her rank, initialed, and handed over to police or put into locked storage, they would stay within Alexandra's sight so that there could be no tampering.

If she did hand them over to someone, she would make sure that he signed off on whatever he was given, including time, his name, date, and his department. This procedure helps forensic nurses collect a higher standard of evidence, something both the police and crime labs appreciate. It makes their job that much easier and also increases convictions. Faced with the knowledge a SANE was doing the rape evidentiary exam, many perpetrators confess on the spot.

Judging from the way the girl grimaced as she was being examined, the nurse suspected hidden bruises.

Turning off the light, Alexandra swept an alternative light source from Omnichrome over the girl's body. Shining in the dark, it picked up secretions on clothing and on skin, showing where both semen and other bodily fluids had been.

Considering that Omnichromes cost $18,000-plus, it had been a fight to get the hospital to pick up the cost, especially because the hospital made no money from these forensic exams.

Since it had been over twenty-four hours since the reported event, in all likelihood bruising had started to occur. Because Marilyn was African-American, her skin did not show bruising as clearly as a Caucasian's might. Most of the bruises could not be seen with the naked eye, but with the light penetrating the first layer of skin, Alexandra could see the marks. With a special camera, the nurse photographed what the light source showed.

"Where else do you have pain?" Alexandra asked.

Marilyn pointed to her side.

Sweeping the light over that area, Alexandra could see three fingerprints clearly on the skin, though they had not been visible with the normal light.

These would be harder to photograph, but she could measure them and determine the approximate size of the offender's hand. This was validation of the victim's story.

Alexandra also lit up the area between Marilyn's inner thighs, where the assailant might have used his hands to push her legs apart and perhaps hold them. She used a variation of the black light here and realized that without her SANE training she would not have even thought to look here. Even though her light wasn't as strong as the one the police would use, it was enough. There were fingerprints there. On her SART report, the nurse marked all the places where questionable areas appeared.

This, Alexandra thought, was good corroborating evidence, but unless she took photos, the case would probably not go to court.

Several times during the initial exam, Marilyn was asked if she would like the nurse to call in the rape advocate.

Marilyn wasn't ready yet.

Alexandra then took swabs of all the areas, including inside the vaginal vault. She had learned that sometimes sperm could remain there up to five days. Not all states do the process of swabbing, but it can help to get more evidence.

As a SANE, Alexandra had to remain totally objective in her care of the patient, noting only items that could be effective in proving or disproving what they suspected had happened. She could not appear to be biased in any way. If the case ever went to court, the defense attorney would sniff out any bias on the nurse's part with the ferocity of a hunter dog.

The rape advocate, often an unpaid volunteer, can be there with the patient, hold her hand, guide her through the legal and medical systems, and keep her from getting upset. It isn't unusual for a victim to have what Dr. Ann Burgess, a Ph.D. of nursing, dubbed rape trauma syndrome. This includes nightmares, depression, low self-esteem, and numerous other difficulties in readjusting to normal life. The rape advocate is there to stand by the victim and make sure she receives proper treatment. The rape advocate has the liberty to believe everything and anything the victim says without question, whereas the nurse has to find evidence to support any fact she states in her reports.

Continuing the exam, Alexandra explored the victim's genital area—both exterior and interior areas of the vagina and anus. Combing the pubic hair onto a clean sheet of paper, the nurse checked for anything foreign or unusual. Several hairs had clumped together near the opening.

Since many rapists in this modern age of DNA are savvy enough to use condoms, sperm is often not found inside the vagina. But sometimes it spills over into the pubic hair or the inner thighs.

The rape evidence kit provided swabs and other material with which to take and preserve specimens, but there was none for pubic hair. Since Alexandra knew there could easily be semen or some other bodily fluid on the hair, she snipped off the strands, folded them into a piece of clean white paper, and sealed it into an envelope. Then she wrote on the envelope what the contents were, where she had found them, the time, date, her name, and the necessary identification of the patient. (Only someone skilled in sexual assault exams would have included these possibly telltale hairs.)

For the internal exam, Alexandra used the colposcope. If the machine's magnification, which enlarged the view 250 times, picked up anything worth noting, she would use the camera to add it to the evidence.

Alexandra photographed a slight redness at the mouth of the woman's cervix, even though this might be the result of a normal sexual encounter. However, Marilyn told the nurse this was her first sexual experience. Even in this day, when casual sexual intercourse was much more prevalent, Alexandra saw no reason to disbelieve her.

The hymen showed neither tearing nor anything else abnormal. Old wives' tales used to attribute the rupture of a hymen to horseback riding or to a girl or woman's first sexual experience. (Later, tampons were added to the list). Alexandra recalled hearing about wedding-night sheets soaked with blood. The physiological truth is that the hymen is not a solid membrane. Yet even though she was a nurse, until she had taken the SANE training, Alexandra herself had believed the tales. Actually, the hymen is similar to an elastic hairband that expands to capture whatever it encircles. The degree to which it can stretch depends on how much estrogen the woman's body is producing. All through the years of menstruation, unless there are hormonal problems, and until late into menopause, the hymen remains easily elastic, expanding and contracting as needed.

Blunt-force injury with a foreign object (including an erect penis or such harmful instruments as a Coke bottle or baseball bat) can and often does rupture the hymen and cause tearing or tags, but the normal hymen does not need to rupture with sex. It already provides an opening in order to release menses.

In an attempt to catch any minute injuries that she had not been able to see even with magnification, the nurse stained the area with a blue dye that would be absorbed by injured tissue while that on unhurt tissue would wash away. But nothing showed.

Of course, she could always have the young woman return for a follow-up visit in a few days in case more of the internal bruising was evident then. But the time to persuade Marilyn to decide whether or not to make a police report was now.

All during the exam, something had been nagging at Alexandra, some idea that she couldn't bring up in her conscious mind.

"Did you find something?" the patient asked.

"It's hard to say. In the meantime, I would very much like for you to call in a report, but you have to make that decision yourself. Perhaps you'd like me to call the rape advocate first and you can talk about it with her."

"I don't know." The girl hesitated. "Maybe I should ask the doctor?"

Alexandra did not want to put the doctor down, but she knew that most doctors had little or no experience with, or interest in, the trauma of rape unless it involved physical wounds that they could treat.

"Sure," the nurse said. "I'll get him." Without leaving the patient or the evidence, which she had collected without a witness, she went to the desk and had the doctor on call paged. It took a half hour for him to appear.

Taking the physician aside, Alexandra gave him a brief history of the event from the patient's perspective and a list of her own findings.

"You did the pelvic, nurse?" His brow rose.

"Yes, I did a pelvic exam to look for trauma, doctor. I did not look for anything but the trauma," she said, trying to remain pleasant. Was it only that he didn't want to be involved or was he really ignorant of what sexual assault was? He had never wanted to do rape exams before. Was he really upset that Alexandra has done this one?

"I'm sorry, nurse, but you are overstepping your boundaries. And why is the colposcope in place? Surely you didn't use that, too?"

Alexandra closed her eyes for just a moment to think of a reply that would not be too rude. "Doctor, I did not do colposcopy. I used the colposcope for seeing the trauma."

"So you saw trauma."

"No." Alex sighed. "I saw no internal trauma, doctor, except for the redness by the cervical os."

"Which, as we know, can be any number of things, including consensual sex. Right?"

Alex flushed. "Correct. But there is plenty of evidence of bruising. Doctor, if you would like to do the complete exam, it only takes about three to four hours . . ."

"Three hours? You have to be kidding."

"Three hours, at least, doctor. If you wish, I am happy to release the patient to your care. But then, of course, you will be the one called into court should there be any questions." She handed him the multipage OCJ forms that needed to be filled out for any sexual assault reported.

"Doctor, I think you'll find a column addressing your concerns in the *Journal of Emergency Nursing*. We only do pelvics for the purpose of the rape exams. We do not look for cancer or other abnormalities. We only use the colposcope for taking evidentiary photos and exploring for trauma that we cannot see with the naked eye. I'll put the article on your desk, too."

The doctor rolled his eyes.

"If you're quite ready, doctor, let me show you what I have found."

She told the patient that she was going to turn off the light and use the Omnichrome again.

"Hmm. Hmm," the doctor repeated several times. "Had some rough sex, did we, dearie? Into S & M, maybe?" He looked at the bruises on her wrists.

Then the physician glanced at his ER chart. "When *was* the last time you had sexual intercourse, Marilyn?"

"Doctor, I told you. Marilyn told me she is a virgin."

The doctor rolled his eyes. "Nurse, you forget this is a college town. The only virgins here are the ones under the age of twelve, and even then . . ." He left the sentence hanging.

To Marilyn, he said, "Are you sure you didn't just have a problem with your boyfriend?"

The patient looked as if she was about to burst into tears. "I . . . I don't have a boyfriend. I am . . . I was . . . a virgin. Am I still?" She looked first to the doctor and then the nurse.

"Of course . . ." the doctor started.

". . . you are," the nurse finished. "Marilyn, I am going to call the rape advocate for you. She's just down the street. So it won't take long for her to get here. And then . . . You can decide if we call the police."

"I . . ."

"Nurse, if there is no trauma, then there was no rape."

"Doctor, just because there are no physical findings doesn't mean rape did not occur. In this case, we have bruising, especially on her inner legs and her breasts, where I have taken swabs. We also have redness of the cervix and possible bodily fluids on the pubic hair. I think we have a case. I would like her to make a police report, but the choice has to be hers."

He didn't even hear her. "I'll give her the usual for STDs and pregnancy prevention." He signed the chart with an egotistical flourish. "Now I have to see patients who really need me."

The nurse was obliged to notify the police of the events of the night. But the victim did not have to talk to the police if she did not want to. "It's within your civil rights not to speak of the matter. But I hope you will. It could help us to get someone dangerous where he can't hurt anyone else. You survived. The next girl might not be so lucky."

Finally the patient agreed that seeing the police was the best thing.

It didn't take long for the detectives to arrive. Once again, the nurse went with them over her chart and the specimens she had taken. She had called the rape advocate, who arrived as well, and so, with the multidisciplinary team in the room, the patient once more told whatever she could recall of the events of the night before.

Alexandra was glad that everyone had come together. It was often hard for the patient to keep repeating the story over and over. Even when going over the same ground, the victim will sometimes recall different things and sometimes forget other points. This makes her look as if she is fabricating or adding elements, when, in fact, the victim of rape trauma syndrome often finds some things become more clear as she rehashes the events.

As Alexandra was finishing her notes and signing over the evidence to the police, she recalled what it was that had kept nagging at her. Just a month earlier she had had another case and done the exam of that victim. The details had been similar, but that party had been at one of the local frat houses.

The exam had shown similar mild injuries— external bruising and redness but no actual tears or real injury seen. The victim had also been unable to recall the events. Only with that case, there had been no indication of possible bodily fluids trapped in the hairs.

She was glad that the girl had finally agreed to talk to the police. It was easier for them to make a case with Marilyn's participation. Even though she didn't believe she knew much, her body—the crime scene—had testified for her.

Alexandra mentioned the previous case to the police, who told her that they still had no leads on that case and agreed to check into it to see if there were similarities. Since the grass roots organizations have made police more aware of rape, it was rare in a city of this size that they would ignore any complaint.

Although it took several months for all the tests and the investigation to be completed, the DNA from the hairs taken from Marilyn matched that in the saliva swabbed off the first rape victim and yet a third girl. The perpetrator, a senior in the frat house where the first party had occurred, pleaded innocent until he realized what evidence they had on him. The SANE's dedication and powers of observation had stopped a serial rapist.

In some areas, a prescription drug from the same family as Valium, Xanax, Halcion, and Librium is known as a "rape drug." It is not sold legally in the United States, but it's available here, and in other countries it is legitimate, prescribed for sleeping disorders. Its street name is "pappas," or "potatoes." The drug is a kind of Mickey Finn, making the person who takes it unconscious and unable to remember what happened. Both it and Valium are sold illegally to be slipped into drinks in order to knock the drinker out.

As a forensic nurse, Alexandra had also examined suspects brought in by the police. It was important, when examining these people, to keep an open mind, collecting only evidence that could be tested and that would stand up in court. She had to keep in mind that to be accused is not the same as being found guilty. There are safeguards for everyone, not just for the seemingly innocent.

More than once Alexandra had been able to prove that the man brought in as a suspect was actually innocent of the crime of which he had been accused.

＊ ＊ ＊

SANE's forensic training in that city has been a significant factor in providing the evidence to prove suspects innocent or guilty. Since the SANEs had started their forensic exams, the prosecution of cases had gone way up. When, for budget reasons, the sexual assault response team they worked for (headed not by a forensic nurse but by a nonmedical administrator) wanted to return to using residents and doctors for their exams, the DA refused to allow that. Not only that, it was easier to bring the nurses to court, he said, but the random residents who frequent the ER on an irregular basis are difficult to find a year or two later when the case is heard. Often, when they are found, they are loath to attend the trial.

In the course of their forensic examinations of victims of crime, SANEs have often provided the evidence that not only helped to convict a criminal, but in many cases led to the perpetrator's arrest and conviction.

On the night of October 4, 1997, twenty-one-year-old Amber, a prostitute, stood on a San Francisco street corner looking for trade. A white Cadillac pulled up and the driver offered her $150 for her services. Needing clothes for her child, she agreed and got into the car.

What she didn't know was that the man, a plumbing contractor named Jack, was free on bail from three earlier sexual assault cases, including that of a former girlfriend. He had a criminal history dating back to the sixties and including five prison terms and a recent assault on another prostitute. Yet he was also a man who liked Chopin and Rachmaninoff, and who quoted Camus and Sartre.

More than one acquaintance claimed he could "charm the pants off a rat." He chose to assault prostitutes because he believed, as did many others, that they were safe victims: Their credibility was often in question due to their profession, and if they accused him, they would not be believed.

With Amber in the car, he drove to an area off Bayshore Boulevard. There he tied her hands with telephone cord and raped her twice. Eventually, he forced her from his car, telling her he loved her and asking her if she loved him.

"Yes," she said, petrified for her life. "Yes."

Forcing her head between her legs, Jack began beating her with what she told the nurse she thought was a hammer. "My head pounded. It sounded like an egg cracking." Blood gushed from her wounds. Putting her back in the car, he wrapped her in a plastic garbage bag like a sack of potatoes, stopped at a car wash, and doused her with water.

She bit through the plastic in two places in order to breathe, then collapsed, remaining as motionless as she could. She hoped he would think her dead and leave her or "throw her against a garbage can, like they did in the movies." But he didn't.

Instead, he drove to Pier 9, pulled her out of the car, and threw her, still tied in the bag, over the Embarcadero into the freezing bay.

She waited what seemed like an interminable time, hoping that he had not stayed around to watch her drown, then, dizzy with the blood loss, she clawed her way out of the bag, swam to shore, climbed over a fence, and hailed a passing motorist.

At the hospital, the forensic nurse team got to work. The victim's body was the crime scene and, as such, told the story without her having to say a word.

Semen had been washed away but, as the SANE said, there was still plenty of other evidence to find despite her tumble into the bay.

Her skull bore round indentations left by the blows of the hammer. The SANEs were able to take photographs of the evidence and, with their help in identifying the patterned injury, the police were able to discover the weapon used and trace it back to Jack.

Traditionally, prostitutes are loath to complain to the police, because they fear being arrested themselves or not being believed. Many a hardened cop or attorney just assumes that prostitutes are lying. But the forensic evidence, the silent language of the crime, will be there to verify their attacks even without their speaking of it.

Jack faced forty charges in connection with a string of attacks on four women dating back to 1993.

Not all the charges were substantiated, but thanks to the help of the five SANEs who had treated most of his victims, facts and pieces were put together to build a case. The DA was pleased and, just recently, Jack was sentenced to sixty years. They suspect that he killed and injured many more people than they have accounted for, and they are glad to get him off the streets.

Col. Robert Ressler of FBI profiling fame has said, "Often the best way to approach a profile is through the victimology," i.e., looking at the victim's background. The SANE who sees the victim and talks to him or her at length sometimes can provide the key to a case.

"The more I talk with the patient, and the more at ease she becomes, the more I learn," one SANE told me. "Often I hear things that the cops don't know. The victims tell me things that they think they might have told the police but they have forgotten just what they said and did not say.

"By the time I have finished the exam, a good three to six hours, the victim and I are on first-name basis. I tell her, I know you have already told this to the police but I am charting this. I will be going to court on what you say and what I write. I want to understand it exactly as it happened. So I need to ask you a few more questions. This is what my testimony is based on.

"After I said that, this one girl told me about how the rapist used an old T-shirt to wipe off his penis. He had thrown it into the bushes near the river edge where the incident had occurred. She hadn't mentioned this to the cops because she was so shocked and frightened about the events that she had forgotten about the old T-shirt until we began talking about the rape.

"I told the detectives afterward about the T-shirt. They hadn't known about it. They were able to go back to the scene, find the shirt just where she said it would be. After testing it for the sperm, they were able to make an arrest."

If the nurse does not know how to talk to the patient, she will not hear what the patient is saying either vocally or silently. It's important that we talk to them in their vocabulary. Many people don't know the word "sodomized," but they can relate to "Did he put his penis in your butt?"

What do negative results really mean? What does it mean when we don't find sperm? Does it mean the woman was not raped? Does it mean it happened so long ago that our evidence is lost?

The SANE needs to think beyond the actual insertion and sex act. What type of evidence can she find besides the genital injuries?

In a long-term care facility, Martha, an eighty-year-old Alzheimer's patient, often cried out in her sleep; the staff attributed it to dreams—or nightmares. She would say that her husband, long dead, was in her room, kissing her and making love to her. None of the staff paid much attention. After all, she was old. She was senile.

This scenario went on for nearly three years. But one day, Cora, one of the kitchen helpers, delivering a lunch tray, heard her crying out. She thought she also heard the voice of one of the male LVNs (licensed vocational nurses) coming from the room. Martha was pleading, "Help! Help me!"

Cora knocked loudly. "Are you all right, Martha? Martha?" she called. "Thomas?"

Almost immediately the door swung open. "Yes, Cora. Ah, lunch." He smiled at the kitchen helper. "I was just helping Martha to dress."

Still uneasy, Cora left the room. Something was not right. She bent to pick up a crumpled tissue near the bed.

She stopped at the nursing station and waited patiently for the head nurse to get off the phone.

"Yes, Cora?"

"Something's not right. Miss Martha is . . ."

"Okay. Okay, Cora. I'll go check." She stood, not even letting the kitchen helper finish her sentence.

This, Cora knew, was not going to work.

Back in the kitchen, she asked the others if they had seen anything strange around Martha's room.

One of the other kitchen workers recalled that a few weeks before, the room to another patient's door had been locked. This patient, a new arrival, also was senile. And she, too, had told the staff that her husband had come to visit her the night before. Unfortunately, the staff had not known if anyone had been in the locked room with her.

Cora waited a few more days, wondering what to do. She had no proof of anything wrong but it still seemed strange.

Nearly a week after the incident, Cora happened to arrive at the nursing station just as the day shift was reporting off. She cornered the director, who frowned and took some notes. Thomas was not working that day.

The director wanted an investigation started but needed first to talk with Martha's son for permission. Then she called in a SANE to see the patient. Vaginal swelling was discovered. The SANE told her that sexual contact could have taken place but without doing the tests for sperm, etc., they would not know.

"Sorry," the district attorney told the director when he called, "but that isn't enough for me to set a case on. She might just have an infection." It looked like Thomas was off the hook.

Because Martha had not been able to give a history of any wrongdoing, the SANE had only checked her vaginal area, which seemed the most likely for any sexual misconduct. She realized that not only had they not done a rectal check but also they had not done proper swabs of the other parasexual areas.

The following day, the SANE called the director and asked if Martha could be brought back to the exam area.

The SANE was not surprised to find some serious anal tears.

"Do you think he did it?" the DA asked. "How can we get him?"

Cora recalled the tissue in her pocket and handed it over to the lab. But there was no semen present. The donor of the fluids on the tissue had, tests revealed, a vasectomy. As had Thomas. But there was still no proof. Thomas acknowledged the tissue but said he had a cold that day and had spit into the tissue.

If the SANE could not come up with anything more positive, they would have to release the guy, the DA told the director, since the LVN did not meet any of their profiles and there was nothing on the tissue that could hold him.

The SANE thought about the sexual act and thought about foreplay. Even though Martha had not been a willing partner in all this, some rapists, in what is called "power reassurance," like to fool themselves into believing that their actions are encouraged and even wanted. They fantasize that this is a true relationship of equals. They will often engage in foreplay, because it then feels like the sexual act is a normal culmination.

On that chance, the SANE took swabs of the breast areas, where during foreplay a man might suckle, as well as the inner thigh area, looking for remnants of saliva. The SANE asked to test Thomas's saliva.

The DNA came back a positive match.

Thomas, it was discovered, had gotten his job with forged papers. He had several aliases, and under two of those had been arrested in other states for sexual misconduct with patients in homes where he had worked. Two other names he used were under suspicion.

Like Martha, those who cannot speak for themselves are often the easiest victims and the hardest cases to prosecute. Often SANEs are called in to inpatient mental health units to assess a potential victim. Sometimes the person's capability to consent to the exam presents a problem. Consent is needed for either a sexual assault exam or for a report of criminal sexual conduct.

In these instances, the SANE must turn to psychiatry to determine if the person has enough reasoning skills to understand the nature and purpose of the exam and proposed treatment and the consequences of lack of treatment. If the patient is found incapable, consent from his or her legal guardian is needed.

On September 27, 1997, at two a.m., forty-year-old Hannah came into the ER of a large teaching hospital saying that someone she knew had raped her. More than half rape victims are assaulted by someone they know. These are not always cases of "date rape," where the assailant thinks he is "owed" it for an evening on the town, or believes the woman has been "leading him on." Often the degree of acquaintanceship can be very slight—a "hello" to someone in the elevator, a nod to the grocery delivery boy.

Julie, the SANE on duty the night Hannah came in, collected the evidence as instructed and did a genital exam using the colposcope both before and after dyeing the area with a special blue dye.

She started at the top and worked down, checking for oral, vaginal, and rectal evidence. The rest of the exam and the documentation of body injuries she left for later, since she was anxious to get the evidential swabs and air-dry them as quickly as possible.

The victim had already been medically cleared, outside of the injuries resulting from the sexual assault.

The nurse noticed redness and a tear on one of the vaginal lips. Redness in a bodily area usually means an increased blood flow caused by an injury to that area, possibly made by hitting, slapping, or pounding. There was also redness on the cervix and posterior.

Applying the blue dye, the SANE noted a positive uptake, signifying a fresh injury, and the speculum exam revealed tiny red measles-like spots called petechiae on the patient's cervix as well as some minimal bleeding at the mouth of the cervix. The presence of petechiae also indicated the lack of oxygen that accompanied a pounding or bruising injury. There was clear indication here of nonconsensual sex.

As was her custom, the SANE took colposcopic photos of the injuries and charted her findings.

Despite positive identification of the perpetrator, the case did not go to trial until May 13, 1998. The defendant was charged with second-degree rape.

Often perps who are smart realize that with today's sophisticated equipment and lab tests, their DNA will be discovered, which will place them at the scene. They plead consensual sex rather than claim that they were not there at all.

At the pretrial hearing, the defendant's lawyer presented photographs showing a metal ring worn on his client's penis. He argued that the injury sustained by the woman could have been made during consensual sex. The victim had stated there had been no ring there at the time of the assault. It was the SANE, however, who made it very clear that even if the ring had been present, its clasp—the only part that could have caused the injury—was *opposite* the injured spot. And she had photos of her own that proved it.

It took only two hours for the jury to return with a guilty verdict.

This case represented the first successful prosecution of an acquaintance rape case in that county. Understanding the mechanism of injury played an important role in the examination of this victim, as it does in every instance. The SANE's expertise in interpreting the patterned injury helped to convict one more rapist.

Even though FNs are trained on how to testify in court, it is still an unnerving experience, especially our first experience.

Having watched *Perry Mason, Matlock,* and all the judicial series, I had fully expected for the defense attorney to question me on my own vulnerabilities. After all, he had to discredit my testimony and me as much as he could. Yet to my surprise, I was asked very few questions about my own "victimization" and my own "hatred of men."

It's true that we can be asked almost anything in court, but do we have to answer everything? Absolutely not, according to one DA. A good prosecutor should listen to all the questions, be ready, pencil poised, to object, should the defense ask something untoward.

In a class on courtroom communication, we learned how to best present ourselves in court, how to pause for effect in our presentation of the facts, how to avoid giving opinions unless we are asked as expert witnesses, and how to talk to the jury. As nurses we are trained to interpret medical material to lay people. We also learned that the defense attorney, even though we might not like what he is doing at that moment, is only doing his job. He is trying to get his client freed and that means anything in his power, even if it comes to attempted discreditation of the witness.

As SANEs we can be one of two witnesses: either an expert witness, which means that based on our specialized, advanced skills and our experience, we have expertise that we have developed over many exams; or as a fact witness, which means that we simply state the facts of injury as we see them.

As expert witnesses, once the court qualifies us, we can state our opinions as to the cause of injury and make judgment calls that others are not qualified to do.

As fact witnesses, again, "we only state 'em as we see 'em."

Since nurses are thought to be so empathetic and sympathetic, we are often the one whom the victim tells the events to. We hear what is called by the police a "fresh complaint." That means we are the first to be told the complaint.

As a result of this, we are sometimes privy to information that she has not told the police. It is our job to make sure the police have all the facts at hand.

No matter if we are fact or expert, we are testifying not for the victim, not for the defense, but for justice. For this reason, and for our credibility in court and elsewhere.

DAs, as Henrico County's Sherry Will from the Virginia Commonwealth Attorney's Office, are so supportive of the SART program and the SANE that they offered willingly to have other DAs speak with them.

Not all DAs spend the time needed to speak with the SANE before her testimony, though it was found that those who did ended up with a higher percentage of successful prosecutions.

During the pretrial discussion, one important facet is what the SANE has learned during the exam. A good DA will work with her and prepare the types of questions that would most likely elicit the information the nurse needs the jury to hear. Often the DA himself, who might only have sketchy medical information, needs to be taught the basics of human sexuality.

After all, if we, nurses, fell for the closed hymen = virgin myth, think about the other educated people who have also.

The ability to see past one crime and link it to a pattern is called linkage blindness, yet another way that the forensic nurses can help the police.

Tammy had been working nights as a waitress at a local bar. The last one to leave one Saturday night, she was accosted near her car and dragged into an alley, where an unknown assailant raped her.

Fearing for her life, she had gone along with the

stranger's commands and was relieved when he let her go.

Believing herself unhurt except for her psyche, Tammy did not go to the ER and did not report the rape for several days. She was afraid that her boyfriend would think the assault was her fault and that he would have nothing more to do with her, especially since he had several times asked her to quit working at this bar. Besides, she had been wearing her sexy black skirt and low-cut top, the outfit all the waitresses at this bar wore.

Several days later, the itching started. The urge to scratch got so bad Tammy could think of nothing else. At least that distracted her from her depression for a short while.

Unable to go to work, unable to do much of anything, she finally decided she had to go to the ER. She still had not talked to her boyfriend, nor had she told any of her friends about the rape.

Paula, the SANE working that night, also worked in a family practice clinic by day. She immediately recognized the severe itching and reddish-brown "dust" in the patient's underwear as being caused by crabs, or the crab louse.

After taking time to explain what was going on, and performing the initial exam, Paula had won Tammy's trust. She told the girl that crabs were mainly transmitted by sexual contact and that they localized in the genital region. Often they were accompanied by other forms of sexually transmitted diseases. Since venereal disease was a possibility, the nurse needed to know whom else Tammy had intercourse with.

Then the young woman opened up and told the nurse about her frightening experience.

Since the SANEs of that area had weekly debriefings to talk about their cases and make sure that they were doing all they could for their patients, Paula recalled that just the week before there had been another rape, and the victim, who also had blond hair and worked in a bar, but one across town, had come down with crabs.

After a short discussion, Tammy finally agreed to make a report to the police.

As the detectives were leaving, Paula told them about the other case. "Would you like me to check our records at the family clinic and see if anyone there is reporting crabs, too?"

The detectives agreed that it was an excellent idea and asked her if she could check with some of the other clinics for them, since she had the rapport with the staff and could talk their language.

It wasn't long before the rapist was caught and identified. He had, in fact, been a patient at Paula's clinic.

Jennifer, a blond, twenty-five-year-old graphic artist, was attacked in the parking lot as she was leaving work after a late-night deadline. She was thrown against the hood so that she could not move. Something pressed into her skin. It wasn't sharp, like a knife, more like a bump.

Driving her into a deserted spot near the river, her assailant tortured her and assaulted her, but when he was done, he drove her back to the parking lot and handcuffed her to the door of her car.

Busy with fighting for her life and her dignity, she didn't even really think about the thing pressing into her until much later when she showed up at the emergency room. There had been plenty of injuries for Sue, the SANE, to document, but she wasn't sure if any of the DNA evidence would show anything.

Jennifer's thoughts kept returning to the uncomfortable sensation when he had first attacked her and pinned her arms behind her. "It was hard. But it was metal . . . not . . . uhm . . . you know." The victim flushed. "I think maybe it was a belt buckle or something. You know, one of those ornate ones, like the motorcycle guys wear," she said, referring to some of the metal-worked buckles.

Sue had seen those at a swap meet just the other day. "The ones with the names engraved in raised letters?"

"Kind of. I guess. I don't know."

"Okay." Sue noted it on her report.

Then she finished filing her reports and didn't think a whole lot about the story until she handed the paperwork over to the detective in charge of the case.

At the peer case review held the following Sunday, where several of the local SANEs from the Sexual Assault Investigators group came together, the conversation suddenly took a turn toward weekend plans.

"I'm going to a swap meet," Sue's friend said.

"A swap meet?"

"Yeah. I promised my boyfriend I would buy him one of those name buckles. The engraved ones. Want to come along?"

"Uh, maybe. You know, one of my clients thinks a rapist that attacked her last week was wearing a belt buckle like that." She poured herself some coffee and took her seat as they waited for the next speaker to present her cases.

"Most of those are handmade. A lot of those motorcycle guys work with metal and leather. They sell their wares at the swap meet."

"I know," Sue said. "Well, Detective F. knows about it. I'm sure he'll make the connection."

The women started to talk about something else when the lights flickered for the speaker.

To Sue's amazement, the case that the speaker talked about involved a belt buckle. The assailant had pressed so hard against the victim that part of his name, a D and Y, were clearly imprinted on the victim's skin.

Although this case had happened in a jurisdiction different from the one where Sue worked, she thought the information significant enough to contact the detective with whom she had filed Jennifer's report.

There were even more similarities. Both victims were blond, with long hair; both were artists and attacked late at night, driven to a riverfront spot. Either the assailant, if he was the same one, was becoming cocksure of himself or had forgotten himself in his "passion," for he had not worn a condom during the second attack as he had during the first.

The detective said he would look into the other case, and the speaker also gave her the name of the law enforcement contact in Jennifer's case.

"You would think that they would communicate with each other like we do," Sue told her friend as they drove home.

"But they often don't. They have no real mechanism for talking to one another. Unless something sticks out, they seldom connect the dots."

"Wait," Sue said as she turned the radio on a bit louder.

There was news about an assault, the victim having been taken to a riverfront park upstate, where she was attacked.

Immediately, Sue got her car phone out and called her detective associate again. "I think your fellow struck again in River Heights."

Although she was never formally acknowledged, the detective knew that it was the nurse who had assisted in putting these puzzle pieces of victimology and MO together to help him make the arrest.

Because SANE know that they have to look beyond the obvious, they often follow their own gut instincts in doing exams, especially when, in the aftermath of the assault, the victim has panicked and has trouble recalling exactly the sequence of what happened.

Sometimes the sequence of the acts or the words

that the offender has said or forced the victim to say, can help identify him, if that is his "signature." This sequence of certain acts and/or words is not necessary for him to perform his assault on the victim, but he may be compelled to do things a certain way, making the fact uniquely his. Forensic observers are "leaving his signature," much as, when we sign our names, that extra flourish at the end is not needed to make our names legal on a document, yet we do it anyway.

During their coursework, SANEs deal with the basic human sexual response, which gives them basis for some of their exam ideas. Sometimes the SANE has to try and put herself into the offender's shoes for just a moment. As she listens to the recital of the events, she figures out where to look for clues on the body of the victim.

"Most people forget about the possibility of oral sex," says Carol, a SANE. "They don't look closely at the mouth for trauma as a result of oral sex, but it's often there." She described a case she had had recently.

A young girl had been assaulted in her parents' home by an older friend of the family. The parents had come home early from the night out and found their friend, who had been baby-sitting, naked, standing over their daughter.

Calling authorities immediately, the parents had been panicked about vaginal penetration. No one, except Carol, the SANE on call, thought to check the inner aspect of the lip, where the frenulum connected the lip to the gums. In a case of forced oral sex, Carol knew, the frenulum would rub against the teeth and perhaps show some injury.

If there is just an oral assault, this might be the only physical evidence that can be found. In that case, it was well within the six-hour limit for collecting oral evidence, but even if the time had passed, the nurse would still have been able to identify the injury and tell the court that, in all likelihood, it occurred this way.

In this case, there was no penetration (much to the parents' relief), but there were indications of oral sex. The parents had, at first, objected to the girl's T-shirt being kept for evidence, until Carol explained to them that if semen had spilled onto the shirt, they might be able to find sperm and/or DNA to help with the conviction.

Additionally, in this case, there were also petechiae—little measles-like dots—in her eyes and on her face, telling the nurse that, perhaps in his sexual ardor, or, maybe, to prevent her from talking, the offender had also tried to strangle the girl.

In court, Carol faced one of the top defense attorneys in the area. She had to admit that she was a bit nervous, since he had a reputation for chewing witnesses up and spitting them out.

"Tell me, Miss M., do you work for the prosecutor?"

"No, I do not," Carol said.

"Well, you don't work for me. So, do you work for the victim?"

"No," Carol said again.

"Aren't you an advocate?"

"Yes, I am," Carol admitted. "I'm an advocate for the truth."

"Let me rephrase that, Miss M. Aren't you an advocate for the victim?"

Again, Carol shook her head. "No. I advocate for patient care but I am an advocate for the truth."

The defense attorney frowned and continued.

"Tell me, Miss M., based on what you know, can you state for a fact that a rape happened?"

"No, I can't," Carol said, surprising the attorney. "I was not there. I did not witness the event. I can't say for sure anything happened. All I can say is that my findings are consistent with the story given by the victim and with forced oral sex."

Convicted on the three-strike law, this offender was jailed for ninety-nine years.

And that is what forensic nurses do, as Carol told the attorney: report only the facts as they see them. We take seriously the words of Dr. P. C. H. Brouardel, a late-nineteenth-century French medicolegist, who said, "If the law has made you a witness, remain a man of science. You have no victim to avenge, no guilty or innocent person to convict or save. You must bear testimony within the limits of science."

Not only women are sexually assaulted. When Bob, a slender but not effeminate male, came into the ER with vague complaints of stomach and pelvic pain, the doctor didn't quite know what to do. Lucky for Bob, Patty, the SANE, was on call and put the facts together.

"Do you want to talk about anything?" Patty asked as she took his blood pressure and the other usual emergency room vitals.

The young man broke into sobs and told the nurse that he had been assaulted.

"Do you want to file charges? Shall I call the police for you?"

Bob hesitated. He didn't think the police would believe him or be sympathetic, but Patty reassured him that the police who usually came to their emergency room were "pretty decent folks." The evidence Patty found with the anal tears helped to convict the rapist.

One of the SANE's assets is the ability to work as a resource person for whatever problem the victim might have. Even if she doesn't have the answers, she can call upon the social worker who is usually part of the SART team to assist her.

While it is rare that females are the offenders in sexual assault, it does happen. Most of the accounts we have are from the prisons. However, that is not the only venue for the female aggressor.

One mother brought her tween son into the ER because he kept on wetting the bed, complaining of pain, and having infections. On the history taking, it came out that the child often slept in his mom's bed. The nurse called a SANE to look at the abrasions on the boy's penis and she did a further exam. Taking a swab and impression of the area, it was determined to be teeth marks of the mother.

One of the reasons the police and DAs understand the phenomena of rape and the symptoms associated with it a lot better than they used to is what Dr. Ann Burgess and her colleagues did at Boston City Hospital in the 1970s. Gail Lenehen, R.N., E.D.D., was there helping her from the beginning.

As psychiatric nurses, they were free from the usual hassles of the ER and able to concentrate on the psychosocial problems of rape survivors. In the first year of the study, they followed over 140 victims. The psych nurses were the first on-site SANEs, although they were not yet called by that name. As the psychiatric clinical specialists, they could take care of the rape victims with no MI (myocardial infarction or heart attack) waiting for them. They staffed the ER twenty-four hours a day, seven days a week, just waiting for victims so that they could learn. If there were psychiatric patients who needed help, they let the psych resident take care of them.

Because they could not allow themselves to be distracted by the trauma patients, they realized that regular staff nurses from the ER would not fit the bill . . . at least not right at that moment. Staff nurses had too many other responsibilities, and could not give the rape survivor the full attention needed, because, if you worked staff at the emergency room and you had a rape come in, your colleague had to take up the slack while you concentrated on one patient. This created a lot of tension and it was never quite fair to the victim.

Most of the non-emergency SANEs did not want to do the assault exams and were more than happy to allow those with the passion for justice and the "tedious" paperwork to take the three to six hours needed to do a proper exam. Because they lacked the knowledge and feared going to court, the non-SANEs felt uneasy and nervous when they were forced to deal with rape survivors.

And so, the goal of the new group created by Burgess and Lenehen was primary care of the rape victim. While the resident and gynecologist would still be called in for pelvic exams and general medical care of the victims, those of this new group oversaw the primary patient care. It wasn't long before the residents found it much easier to just let the nurses do the pelvic exams, unless, of course, there was something radically wrong. Then the docs would be called in.

Besides doing the actual evidentiary exam, they would do posttrauma counseling for a couple of days or even a few weeks thereafter. They would go with the victims to court and support them, much as today's rape advocate does. Because their work was largely volunteer, their only perks were knowing that they were helping others—and the time off from their regular duties. Of course, they did get straight pay.

They did not start out as rape advocates, and have since learned that it was better for the SANE's credibility not to be an advocate for the patient, but you can't talk to hundreds of patients and hear their stories and not become an advocate.

The nurses often suffer from vicarious traumatiziaton and even experience some of the fear and symptoms, as do their patients.

"This is mankind at his worst," says one SANE. "It needs to be acknowledged that the work is difficult. Sometimes it's nearly impossible to take. If you have enough nurses to back you up you can take a break when things get too tough."

In the early years, SANEs did not pretend to be neutral in court but did the same thing they do now—relate the facts as they see them, without interpretation. Their objectivity was questioned then, but not as much as one might think.

They learned from the victims that the victims—or survivors, as they prefer to be called—got upset when people treated them with the awkwardness one usually reserves for a situation that one, oneself, would have difficulty handling. Following Ann Burgess and her work, the SANEs at Boston City learned how to ask questions compassionately and how to give the survivors the respect they needed to help regain their self-esteem.

Over the years, the SANEs have moved away from counseling the survivors and concentrated more on dealing with purely forensic aspects of the situations.

Boston City Hospital wasn't the first rape crisis center. In fact, there were may be a handful around the country at the time. Like with many an idea whose time had come, the community was becoming more responsive to rape victims. But we were still fighting against a tidal wave of superstition and stereotypes, and each program was reinventing its own wheels. Most of them came to the same conclusions, eventually but not easily. That's one of the reasons why it is so important that the IAFN helps the SANEs to standardize their programs and certify those taking the training.

In the early '90s, *Journal of Emergency Nursing* printed a list of SANE programs. There were only a dozen or so at the time. Linda Ledray, RN, Ph.D., used that list to invite people to Minnesota for the first international meeting. Now, Linda's articles deal with various aspects of the SANE education and new developments in forensic nursing. We need to communicate with other nurses, doctors, police, and, most especially, the crime labs.

In her role as an editor, she is most surprised at the reaction of the doctors who are now complaining that nurses are practicing medicine by doing the pelvic exams and using the colposcope. "We are not doing colposcopy. There is a difference. I never dreamed we would be fighting doctors to see rape patients, especially since they never wanted them to begin with. Now they are suddenly saying that we are taking their patients. They never wanted to go to court, and now they are upset that nurses are getting called in their stead."

The best way to handle this situation, we find, is to

tell the doc, "I would love to have you do this exam . . . the whole six hours of interviewing the patient and doing the evidence collection." Watch how quickly they back out. You'll be lucky if they stay for the first five minutes of the pelvic. For those who still have doctors holding out and complaining that nurses are practicing medicine, Gail Lenehen and Linda Ledray have written a column that answers all the doctors' questions.

Most SANE programs have a policy stating that a patient with specific injuries or preexisting histories— such as genital bleeding, pregnancy, insertion of a foreign object, difficulty breathing, loss of consciousness, or being younger than fourteen—must be seen by a physician before the nurse can do the SANE exam. It is only when a patient is not severely injured that he or she bypasses the triage desk.

The SANE consults the attending physician regarding prophylactic antibiotics, pregnancy prevention, and other orders, and develops a specific patient plan of care.

Because of the success of the SART programs, the length of hospital stay needed for a sexually assaulted patient has been shortened. Most of this is due to nurses becoming familiar with the process and more experienced.

Five years ago, Rene was a clinical nurse specialist in the emergency room. Then she started to explore what it was that we did for rape victims. She began to see how uneven, variable, and unpredictable the treatment was. Mostly it was based on how busy the ER was that day, who was there, and who was willing to do the case. She looked into the protocol for the department and found there was none.

She went to her state capital and asked for guidelines. To her amazement, there were none. Rene set about developing a program with guidelines. "They probably didn't believe I would accomplish anything, so they gave me carte blanche to do something. I did a training video for the whole state. I showed nurses and others how we had to collect the evidence and what had to happen to make the evidence good. Most nurses knew nothing about forensic technique back then. I recognized poor practice and I knew it had to be improved," she says.

"I copied a model that was being used in New England. It hadn't been widely accepted, but the assistant DA for sex crimes told me to go for it. So we developed a pilot program four years ago that called for SANE funding by the Department of Criminal Justice.

"The program was still rough around the edges. I had someone directly out of the nursing school. She knew what rape was but she had never dealt with the forensic aspect of it. There had to be more depth. I subscribed to the *Journal of Forensic Medicine* and read up on child abuse and forensics. Basically, we had to teach ourselves what it was we were lacking, and then we had to find the skills to fill in.

"By the time we had done between sixty and a hundred exams, we had a good basis for teaching. We knew what we were looking for and how to collect the evidence.

"Were we ready yet? Hardly. We trained for adolescent and adult sexual assault but not for pediatrics yet. Kids are our next step. Yet in spite of not knowing much, we knew more than the local doctors at the ER who would come to us and say, 'Can you look at this child for me?'

"Like being thrown into the fire, we had to cook or burn. Informally, we became quasi-experts in what the doctors and other staff did not want to learn. The downside of this was that the MDs and residents did not have the opportunity to understand interview techniques of a victim. They couldn't comprehend how to look for injury or how to magnify and use forensic enhancing dyes and other techniques. They had no concept of where to look for the injury . . . no matter what we tried to tell them, they would only look inside the pelvic area and would almost always forget the external genitalia. Many of the residents weren't even sure how a normal hymen differed from an injured one. They had never really looked at it. It just was not in their training vocabulary, and it was up to us to train them, to show them how to take photos that could be used in court and would show the genital injury.

"Some of the residents didn't even understand the difference between a laceration and a bruise. To them, and to many people, the presence or absence of a hymen was what constituted rape. The lawyers and police also need to be educated about hymens. They will ask us, 'Is her hymen intact?'

"They mistakenly believe that the intact hymen means that the person is a virgin, and so the rape did not occur. To them the condition of the hymen is the determining factor of rape . . . when, in fact, it has little to do with the rape. Of course it can be injured, but it's not a glass to be shattered with sex, as most people seem to think. It's elastic, like a rubber band, and expands to accommodate when it needs to do so.

"Most doctors don't want to take instruction from nurses, no matter how experienced in something we might be, but finally our OB/GYN residents are beginning to respond and asking to be called in to our training.

"They're coming around slowly, though. I have only had one resident sit through the whole exam. She was like a sponge, soaking up the information that I had to give. Maybe it was because she was female and had a different perspective. The other GYN residents didn't even come down when I called them. Another one stayed for only five minutes."

A good number of the SANE training programs have classes in courtroom communication but not all. We need to work with the DA and know how to perfect our testifying. Yes, we can collect the best evidence and identify many injuries but if we are not prepared properly by the DA for the questions that might be asked, if we can't win in court because we are unprepared, then what good does it do us or the victim.

• • •

Because the SANEs come from a wide variety of backgrounds, not just emergency and not just psychiatry, we can learn from one another. We continue to bring different aspects of our learning to our trainings and to the national conferences held every year, enabling us to think differently about sexual activity and the experiences that our clients are subjected to.

A forensic nurse examiner (FNE) has the knowledge to explain human sexuality to the ordinary person and not be embarrassed by referring to proper names for the genitals in public. If a nurse is uncomfortable saying words like "penis," "labia," and "hymen," think how much harder it is for the layperson.

Two sisters, Sasha and Pina, ages twelve and six, respectively, were brought into the ER. We usually only take twelve and up in our SART program, but I wanted to show the pediatric resident how to do the exam, and, since they were together, it seemed like a good start.

I taught the resident how to create rapport with the six-year-old. "She needs to be sitting higher than you or at eye level." So we both sat down on stools, with her on the exam table looking down at us. I gave her a stuffed animal to hold. Most residents stand when they are talking to their patients . . . maybe that's because they have so many and so much to do and they're always in a hurry. This type of interview is something you can't rush.

"You must be in kindergarten. Or is it first grade?" I asked the child, developing our relationship.

She nodded. "First grade." She was quiet. Shy. Such big blue eyes.

"What are you learning?"

"Letters."

"Do you like your teacher?"

She nodded.

"I'm glad. Do you have a bike at home?"

Again a nod.

"Can you teach me to ride? I never learned how."

She grinned, knowing I was joking.

"Tell me, Pina, has anyone ever hurt you or touched you in a way you didn't like?"

Pina was silent for a very long time. We had separated the two girls, because we didn't want them to be looking to each other for answers.

Finally, she nodded.

"Can you tell me about it?"

Just as she started to speak, the resident's pager went off. I shook my head. "Never leave in the midst of a story like this. You'll never get it back to where it was." He shut the pager off. "You need to hear the whole story from the child. You give them your undivided attention."

"Can you tell us what happened? Who touched you, honey?"

The words tumbled out about her grandfather and her uncle.

When it appeared she was done, I told her that we

had one more step to do. We had to look at her and make sure that everything was okay where she went pee and poop. I had talked with the mother already and learned that these were the words the girl used for her private functions. It's always best to speak to the child in the language they understand.

This gave the resident the chance to look at the genitalia, not just use the technique of lateral separation to look at the six-year-old's unestrogenized hymen. The girl had no visible injury.

"How are you going to document this?" I asked him. "How are you going to write what you saw?"

"Intact hymen?" the resident asked.

I shook my head. "You want to describe the hymen, what it looked like: pink, healthy, thin membrane. You want to write that you saw no bruises, or bleeding, or eccymohysis, or discharge. If you only write that she looks like a healthy child, her claim will be dismissed. If she is at risk and we don't see anything today, someone examining her in a few months could see if our words compared to what he saw. If he sees a notch at three p.m., then he would see something is new."

We then went and examined the twelve-year-old.

The young girl was frightened. She was reluctant to show her body to anyone, especially a man.

"I understand your feelings, dear. But if we are to help other children like yourself, we have to learn."

Finally, she agreed. I showed the resident and the attending doctor in the room how to use the colposcope to magnify the area and to take photos for evidence. I then showed them how to use a Foley balloon catheter in the vagina (often used to help drain urine during and after surgery or when there is an impairment in the urinary tract) to visualize the hymen and make sure that it is not injured. This is especially helpful in younger women.

We saw that the hymen was thickening and estrogenized. There was no physical evidence here of assault, but, as I explained to the resident and attending, a molester often grooms the child, getting her to trust him, getting her to accept what he is doing. Slowly he advances on her, getting her to accept just one more step than they feel comfortable with. And when that is done, he goes a bit further.

Following a teenage sexual assault conviction, I went to an emergency medicine presentation in another state. I was especially interested in their program on how to convict a rapist. The doctor presenting described what the examiners did.

Afterward I went up to the physician who was conducting the program. There was not a single nurse practitioner there. I asked her about her findings and how she had come to some of the conclusions.

It turned out that she was the director of a SANE program. What she described was what the FNEs and the SANEs were doing.

In the discussion after, four attending MDs came up to find out how does the physician not lose control over a situation like this. The director of the SANE program explained that the patient is still in the emergency room, not in private sector.

"You will feel somewhat threatened by giving up some of the control, but they are still under your control to sign out and to give meds to, etc. In our community hospital, we do the exam in a private area off to the side of the ER. We welcome the doctors' attendance, but most of them are just too intimidated by it."

I try to teach the police and others what we deal with, that children, and those who have mental-health or drug problems, are probably the most vulnerable. They're the least likely to be believed and the least likely to give a coherent case history.

"Julie, she doesn't change her story. It's been over two hours. What should we do? How do we know what happened?"

"Is she complaining of any pain?" I asked.

"Uhm . . . yeah," he said.

One of the criteria I used was that pain or bleeding at the time of the incident helps to determine if we will find something. "Then I think we need to do an exam."

At the exam, we picked up significant evidence. I still use slides and show the case around to prove that just because the patient is transient or intoxicated, you can't throw the case out. She still needs to, has a right to, have an investigation. The officer finally said, "My God, it could have been my grandma."

We picked up the suspect but the case is still pending.

* * *

Laurie, a fifteen-year-old girl, came into the ER sobbing. Her neck was in such spasms, she couldn't think, eat, or sleep, and none of the over-the-counter drugs had helped.

After calming her down, Ruth, the SANE, proceeded to perform an exam. Something happened when the girl had been out camping with her mother and stepfather, Ruth's SANE antennae told her.

Ruth remembered from her training that the body is the scene of the crime. Even though the usual exam didn't show anything suspicious, there was still a chance of evidence on other parts of the body. If a rape occurred, there might be other trace evidence even if the perp only touched her mouth, perhaps pieces of leaves or grass that could substantiate at least part of the story.

After noticing how very tight the muscles were in Laurie's neck, Ruth also noted some bruises and raw abrasions there. "How did you get those marks? It looks like someone has been beating you about the neck and shoulders?"

The girl shrugged. "I guess." She was teary-eyed again and couldn't talk much. Her throat, she said, was sore.

Ruth took the colposcope and looked in the back of the girl's throat. She could see petechiae in the back and was able to photograph and document it.

With her own background as a rehab nurse, Ruth re-

alized that the girl would have neck tightness and possibly a neck injury.

It eventually came out that Laurie had been forced
to give her stepfather oral sex while her mother slept.
There had been no one else around the campsite. He
had been beating the back of her head and neck to get
her to do this. Her neck was in spasms from the event.

At the grand jury, Ruth was able to explain how the
neck injury occurred. She drew diagrams of the hyper-
extension of the neck muscles, and had photographs of
the redness and petechiae in the mouth.

Most members of juries, even though they are intelligent men and women, have very little knowledge of
what a sexual assault nurse examiner does and how
different she is from the nurse who changes the bedpans and wipes the sweat with the towel. They do not
know how nurses are being used in rape cases, homicide and natural death cases, in workman's comp and
other legal cases.

When Lana was raped by her date, a pro tennis
runaround and the son of a prominent family, an expensive Texan lawyer was brought in to clear the man
of the charges.

He tried to use whatever trick he could to upset
Lisa, the SANE. On the stand for over eight hours of
testimony, she went through plenty of sidebars (paused
explanations) and learned a lot about what she could
and could not say at a trial. She also learned she didn't

have to answer all the questions that he asked, nor did she have to answer to the degree he seemed to want her to. His basic mission was to confuse the jury and discredit her.

"You are a frustrated doctor, aren't you, Miss S.?" the defense attorney said to the nurse on the witness stand. (She had been called not as an expert but merely as a fact witnesses.)

"No." She smiled sweetly. "I am a nurse because I want to be a nurse. I like being a nurse. If I had wanted to be a doctor, I would have gone to medical school."

He shut up for a moment but came back quickly.

"And nurses do . . ." He paused to look around at the jury, making sure that he had caught their attention. "Nurses change beds, bedpans, pass medications, carry out doctors' orders . . . tell me, what else do they do?"

"You make a good point, counselor." She paused. "Yes, that is what nurses used to do. Some nurses are trained to still do just that. But most nurses make nursing decisions and nursing assessments, both physical and psychosocial. We observe for interactions of medications or other difficulties, solve problems for patients. We do care plans and discharge plans. We communicate with the doctors on the patients' behalf, communicate with patients on the doctors' behalf, teach patients what they need to know about their medications and conditions, and some of us even do research, which profoundly affects how medicine and society react to certain issues. Shall I go on?"

The defense attorney stood there, just gaping.

"Some of us even collect evidence, assist detectives with solving crimes by our observation, help to link cases together by our pooled knowledge, read medical records for district attorneys"—she smiled at the DA who had called her in—"and do other things that are shared with the legal and medical profession."

The defense attorney closed his mouth. Lisa closed hers.

He started up again.

"Most of the time you spend helping the prosecution and detectives is, I believe, volunteer, isn't it, Miss S.?"

"I wish it were. But unfortunately, I have bills to pay, too. Granted, I don't get paid as much as I really should for this type of work, but I do get paid."

"If you are so necessary for the investigation, then why aren't you paid more?"

"Good question. Maybe you can take that up for me with the DA." The jury laughed.

When he had recovered from his embarrassment, he asked, "So, what criteria are used in deciding whether to use you or a technician?"

"I believe you answered your own question, counselor. The answer is money. Law enforcement has a budget, too. I don't believe they budgeted for forensic nurses when they first drew up their plan, but future budgets, I am assured, will include us."

"Hmm. Very well, Miss S., since you are such an expert at sex and sexuality, let me ask you this. Just how big is a penis?"

"Do you mean shrunk or extended?"

The jury laughed.

The jury eventually found the young man guilty of rape, and later told the DA that Lisa's testimony was a help in convincing them.

By far the highest percent of victim population is adolescents.

Anita, the blond teenage girl who came into the ER that night, reminded one nurse of her daughter. The same coloring, same build, same innocent disposition, and there but for the grace of God was her little girl.

She had gone to a bar with friends. A freshman in college, she was innocent and naïve. She didn't recall leaving the bar with anyone, but her friends were able to describe the man she left with . . . a stranger to them all. She scarcely remembered anything at all.

After Anita left the bar with the man around two or three a.m., they were stopped by police on a side road. "Something the matter?" Officer Paul, the rookie who pulled up behind the car, asked as he peered inside and saw the young, blond girl passed out on the seat. "Too much to drink?"

The man nodded. It was obvious, even to the rookie, that this guy had done some serious drinking, too. He was suspicious but didn't know what he could do, since the car was not in motion.

"Need a lift anywhere?" the policeman asked.

"Nope." The man grinned. "My roommate's coming with his car to take us back to her place. Gotta get the girl home, ya know."

Just as the officer was about to question the young man further, another car pulled up.

"Officer Paul?"

The rookie turned. It was Sam, one of his high school buddies. "You're the one picking up this fellow and his girlfriend?"

Sam glanced in the car and then slowly nodded. "Guess so."

"She can't walk very well," said the drunken escort.

"Okay, then," Officer Paul said. "Why don't you guys get on your way after you push the car off to the side?"

His friend nodded. Then the three of them helped to put the young girl into the other car. The officer then drove off, never even making a report, since he knew the guy from high school. He made no connection with the rape victim or the assault until the father of the young girl brought her picture to the station.

She came into the ER fourteen hours later, too late to check for GHB or any of the other psychoactive drugs. Her roommate had brought her in. Both of them were distraught.

Anita had been brutally raped, both anally and vaginally. But she had no memory of the events.

In 40 percent of all the cases of anal rape, the offender used a condom. For a while they could not identify the assailant without the sperm until they began using an anoscope.

With use of the anoscope, identification of rectal trauma went up 45 to 76 percent. More than half of those with rectal trauma had other forms of non-rectal physical injury as well. A complete rectal is needed.

"She had bite marks, thirty-two nongenital injuries, and eleven genital injuries. It was very stressful to document and wash every one of these injuries. I had to draw, measure, and photograph them. She was vomiting with the pain. I had to help her get that under control, as well.

The nurse had the hardest time coming to grips with this case. She went back and had to talk with the other SANEs she worked with. She couldn't talk to her husband. He couldn't relate to the situation.

"In total, it was a six-hour exam. We were both exhausted at the end."

The poor girl developed many health problems as a result: genital herpes, a drug reaction to the medication, urinary tract infections (UTI), among others.

"Have you seen this girl? Did you see her the night of Saturday . . . ?" With no suspect in sight the father took his daughter's picture around town.

Officer Paul stopped short. "Hey, yeah, I did. She had a bit too much to drink. I helped put her in a friend's car to take her home. Why?"

"She was raped," the father said.

"You know who did this?" the supervisor asked.

"I don't know her boyfriend, but I do know his friend Sam."

The rookie and his fellow officers from the sex crimes unit made a visit to Sam, who admitted that he had taken the man and the girl not to her house but back to the man's dorm room.

Everything fell into place. The young man was arrested; he had apparently victimized other young women.

This case has yet to come to trial, but the combination of our work, the work of the police, and the parents helped to stop a rapist. Normally we don't allow parents to get involved like this, but Anita's father, in particular, had taken a very positive and active role in finding the perp.

Julie is one of the lucky ones who have been able to make her career as a SANE a full-time position, but it took many hours and lots of work. "I've always been committed to assessing interpersonal violence in the community. People shy away from child abuse and domestic violence issues, but I was in public health before I became a nurse practitioner. I saw firsthand the devastation of domestic abuse, and I have always had the well-being of the whole person at heart in my nursing problem-solving." That's why Julie had gone for a degree in psychology before she even entered nursing school. She soon found that she needed to have a more concrete way of helping people, not just emotional and psychological.

As a family nurse practitioner, she began by assessing domestic violence. "Our area had had an increase in DV cases over the past few years, and that was pretty surprising, since we're a fairly traditional community." As a result, Julie began gathering support for a local SART team.

"Sherry Ardnt (one of the IAFN founders and a respected SANE) was speaking in Nevada. Several of us, including our DA, went. She was so jazzed by what she heard that, in 1994, she and local law enforcement people helped us start the SART team," Julie says.

They quickly formed a working committee and decided to pattern their group after a successful one in Santa Cruz, California. The hospital agreed to buy a colposcope if the DA would run the program and pay the bills. "We were even reimbursed for attending the monthly meetings," Julie says. "We developed a quality assurance program for our SANEs and had mandatory photocolposcopy training. If a nurse did not do a certain number of exams a year, she had to attend an annual update. In addition, every case was reviewed in detail by the coordinator, both for the quality of the photos and for the outcome of the cases as they followed protocol."

This local team coordinated pediatric and adult exams and found that, due to their efforts, more suspects were being apprehended. As a result, they began doing the suspect exams, too. While other teams in nearby communities fell apart, Julie thinks theirs survived due to good interagency collaboration. "It wasn't uncommon for me to get a call from the cops, the hospital, and Children Protective Services all within five minutes of each other about the same case. The strong leadership of the DA also helped."

For many years, Julie's SART office was located in the DA's office. As head of the SART team, she was hired by the Health and Human Services and on loan to the DA. The respect helped her to establish a leadership role in her community and educate people more about violence. As a result, more of their cases went to court, and those that didn't pleaded guilty from the start.

As head of the SART team, Julie was the only full-time person with ten part-timers on staff. The most difficult thing for the other staff was having to work two or more jobs to keep their hand in this. These exams come in waves . . . there may be three in one night and then none for weeks. If you're the only one on call, it really wipes you out.

When not doing exams, Julie trained and recruited other nurses, did quality assurance, held monthly meetings, budgeted the process, signed bills, stocked the hospitals. Her SART team worked out of two different local hospitals. They did not have a dedicated space but took whatever room in the ER was available, moving their equipment from place to place on a setup cart.

After hearing about some of the problems other programs had had, she was pleased with how supportive their doctors were. Her team saved them the horror of four-hour exams and of going to court. The doctors appreciated that.

Julie herself trained the nurses to do pelvics (for injury observation) and held annual pelvic exam training as well.

Julie believes that one of their biggest successes is their rapport with law enforcement. They talk over everything and try to make their interviews patient- or victim-centered. Then they decide if there is evidence and history that is consistent with description of an assault. Because they see Julie and the other SANEs as experts, the police now call upon them with questions outside of the realm of sexual assault.

"They'd start to call me and ask my opinion if an exam should even be done," Julie says. "They would say, this-and-this is the case, and do you think evidence can be found? Usually I would give it a shot, because sometimes evidence survives beyond the arbitrary date or time we have set."

One homicide case was listed "death from head trauma" but the victim was found naked. That was an indication of a possible sexual assault.

Julie's team had done a training at the local academy, and so the police were familiar with what the sexual assault examiners could and could not do. They decided to ask for a SANE.

It was pretty clear that the victim had been battered in the head with an implement. Julie could see the patterning of the weapon. In fact, she pointed out the ridge markings to them, which helped them to identify the weapon used.

Despite the fact that the morgue had the rape evidence kit and could do it themselves, they called in a SANE since they were not used to doing a rape kit collection, and really didn't know what they were looking for or how to gather the needed evidence.

"I could see trauma with my naked eye," Julie said. She used the colposcope and took several photos. The attendant thought Julie was being rather dramatic about the whole matter. But while she was doing the pictures of the injury, she also saw some fibers, which she never would have seen without the magnification of the colposcopy. Julie had to look carefully behind all the hymeneal folds and trauma, but she found the fibers there. Police were able to pick that up and help to place the killer at the scene.

The sexual homicide, it turned out, was part of a string in the countryside. Julie taking the photos and the evidence off the body helped police to identify the suspect and place him at the scene. Even if he said that the sex had been consensual, there was still a matter of homicide.

Strangely enough, at the next medical meeting, Julie asked the county coroner if he knew Dr. H. "I did a case with him just the other day," Julie said, referring to the sexual homicide.

"Oh, yes," the coroner said. "We were just talking about that case. We don't think there is any role for postmortem colposcopy."

That floored me. Sometimes they just don't get it.

* * *

Sometimes it's the little things that stand out in our minds that help to connect one crime to another, one victim to another.

Barbara became interested in forensic nursing after she lost her sister to a robbery attempt by an angry former employee. Shot in the head, she was still alive when taken to the hospital and transferred to ICU. "We could see them working on her, but we weren't allowed in to talk to her, even though they and we knew she might expire at any moment. I didn't like the way my family was treated by the nurses and doctors at the hospital when my sister died. I was working as an aide in the ED [emergency department] at the time. I realized some changes needed to be made and so I went to nursing school," Barbara says.

"If there is a victim in the ER, I let the family in to see them, even if we are doing the resuscitation, since it might be the last time they see them alive. The family needs to know that you are doing everything possible to save them, and if they are shooed out of the room, they don't know that you're not just standing around and doing nothing.

While working as a maternal and child nurse, Barbara was exposed to a lot of domestic violence, sexual assault, and child abuse. "The hospital I worked at didn't want to set up any program. It took ten years before I was able to convince the hospital to do something.

"Working together with Planned Parenthood, we

wrote a grant for $25,000, which we got from the Department of Criminal Justice. The hospital foundation then found a donor to supply the colposcope. We renovated a special room for us and showed the hospital administration what a community service they would be doing."

Barbara and her friend were the only two to start the program. Being on call 24/7 was rough. In nine months they saw fifty cases, several convictions, and felt validated.

"At first law enforcement did not understand what we were doing," Barbara says, "but today they ask our opinion, and our relationship allows us to attend programs offered for the police. We also do programs for them. We often talk to the newly promoted detectives and explain what we do, educating them as to the role of the forensic nurse examiner, how we document, what we document. We are just mediators and we document facts, I tell them. We write down what evidence we find and document the victims' stories to see if they coincide with the evidence.

"Now the police come in and say, 'What do you want us to do?' Most of the time, we can let them go on with their work and we will page them when we are finished with the exam. They like this, since it frees up their time and they don't have to wait around for the doctor, X-rays, etc. If it's a ballistic case or homicide, we take the bullet, label it, sign it, and save it for evidence, processing it through the chain of custody.

"When one of the SANEs is on duty in the ER, and

a rape victim is brought in, she is given that job—the administration willingly releases her from her other duties, since she is trained to take care of it. If there is more than one case coming in, a backup will be called. There is still a reluctance on the part of the others to care for a rape victim, especially when they have not been skilled in the procedure, and even more reluctance to think they might have to go to court."

Since Barbara is now the nurse manager of her ER, she can incorporate the SANE work into her clinical practice. As a diploma school (three-year program) graduate, Barbara has had hands-on experience. She is not petrified at being with the patients; she is not afraid to try new techniques. While there is still some question as to whether a diploma or a university (four-year program) nurse makes the better sexual assault examiner, she feels that passion and willingness to learn are just as important.

"Now the doctors are grateful to have us," she says, "and they become upset when one of us cannot be reached for a case. Our local Planned Parenthood has the rape crisis advocate line.

"Talking to several schools, we have educated teachers about sexual assault and the emergency it causes. Sometimes we meet with reluctance and rejection, sometimes with acceptance.

"We reach out and talk with college students, especially freshmen, about date rape. One of the biggest concerns of college students is that they do not want their parents to know, even though the treatment would be covered under the parents' insurance. It worries me that the students are afraid to talk with their parents, but we have set up payment plans for several of them to pay for the services without their parents knowing.

"At the frat and sorority houses, we have lectures on the signs and symptoms of GHB abuse. They need to know what rape is, and when to come to the ER.

"Now that the SART program is under way, we want to establish a domestic violence program.

"The police now respect us and come quickly when we beep them."

Barbara and her group were ecstatic when the medical examiner invited them to the morgue. One of the police officers had listened to their plans and helped them to expand their services to a new level.

An unidentified female body had been found near the freeway ramp with no clothes on.

"Do you think there could have been a sexual assault?" the ME asked.

"Very possible," Barbara and her cohorts said.

They had never done a rape kit on a dead body before, but with the help of the police and the morgue attendants, they accomplished it and showed them what they did and how to work the colposcope and how to check for semen. Explaining everything they did, Barbara and her colleagues saw and collected the semen, swabbed for other evidence, used the alternate light source, which showed bruises and fingerprint marks, and did the photos that the cops would need for court.

Since then, they have been to the ME's office several times to help collect evidence. Now, if there is any suspicion, they are called in. A body was thrown from a car, half-dressed—but they were able to collect DNA evidence from it.

Barbara has since learned that nurses do care and that they can make a difference in others' lives.

Sandra Goldstein was also among the first seventy-two to join Linda Ledray and Virginia Lynch in Minnesota. Calling herself a SANC (sexual assault nurse clinician), she realized that she did forensic nursing without knowing what it was called.

Because she was a family health nurse, Sandra's first intro into the rape crisis was wanting families to be healthy. "Postpartum was where I worked, and I taught parents how to care for babies. But I was seeing a lot of women and children being victimized." In 1986 she was approached to join the team, and was trained by Dr. Laura Slaughter.

Nurses are judged by how quickly they answer a call bell, warm up a stethoscope, bring ice water, and make beds. They are judged on tasks and not on knowledge. No one, including the doctors or lawyers, seems to understand the depth of information and background of science that nurses have.

A nurse from a two-year program may already have four years of college behind her, which would include early-childhood development, chemistry, microbiology, and physiology. Among these nurses attending the two-year programs, the average age is thirty-five. They have been through life, and they have seen some things.

Most people think of nurses as "sweet young things" or "baggy old things," without realizing how much knowledge of science and critical thinking has to go into any nursing judgment. Coming from a history of charity and volunteer work, the nurses of the past were often homeless women and/or prostitutes who were given shelter and food in exchange for nurturing the sick and taking care of the wounded. The doctors came from a background of priestly knowledge about magic, herbs, and healing.

Using all our nursing knowledge and combining it with criminal justice knowledge just makes us that much more formidable in dealing with perpetrators.

We have nursing skills, which helps us to make nursing diagnoses and follow through with nursing care. But also, since we, as nurses, are mandated reporters of child abuse, domestic violence, elder abuse, and sexual abuse, it would help if in the nursing schools we were routinely taught how to identify these crimes and how to properly document them and work with the law and various agencies to get these offenders.

Three years before, Sandra had read a book about a nurse who had put a rapist in jail with the evidence she collected. That was when she started thinking about what she was doing and how she was doing it.

It was at the first meeting that the IAFN SANEs decided to look at standards for practice and develop a strong national voice. Together with Sherry Ardnt, Sandra joined the California Sexual Assault Investigators Association (CSAIA), which at that time was mainly police and prosecutors.

Since media is the best way to educate the public, nurses have to make it happen for themselves. We need to encourage TV shows to include forensic nurses in their crime-fighting units and incorporate what we do with the law.

Sandra's group started the first newsletter, printed on a copy machine. It was not polished or slick, but it had facts. "The goal was to get the information out any way we could. Nurses wanted information about classes, programs, and tips from the crime labs on what evidence to collect and how to process it."

This would later become the *Journal of Forensic Nursing*, which later still evolved into *On The Edge*, the newsletter for IAFN. Eventually, Sandra would like to see a journal of our own, where a group of peers can review articles. The fact is that every nurse is a forensic nurse in trauma, peds, psych, operating rooms, OB/GYN, and just about anywhere. They just don't think about it in the correct way. We need to change their attitudes and to educate them, so that they join us in the fight for justice.

In nursing school, we are frightened into submission. If we don't chart correctly, if we don't document something right, we will have to go to court. We are told that the defense attorney will chew us up and spit us out. The implication is that we do not have the guts or brains to stand up. Nurses are usually females, and defense attorneys are usually males, so, because they are superior, they will win. Court became something to be feared and not something to help us work with the police toward justice.

Thoughts and attitudes have to change. We had one male nurse who had taken the SANE training, and he was very good. We phoned an OB, who often let our students do preceptorship with him. "I don't think I can precept this guy," he said. "The women are not going to want a man examining them." This is someone who has always been very supportive of our program and of nurses in general. It floored me that he, a man, would say this.

As one of the oldest successful SANE programs, Sandra's group (www.forensicnursing.com) has set up educational guidelines and does five-day intensive trainings with preceptorship set up for those wishing to start a program. And on the Web, or through the mail, Linda Ledray also has guidelines set up for those wanting to start a unit. The step-by-step guides help you through the setup, from dealing with police and DA to the funding and the patients.

"It's exciting how many calls I am getting from nurses who are interested in this new field," Sandra says. " 'How do I get in?' 'Where do I work?' "

Unfortunately, forensic nurses aren't being hired or utilized in as many places as they can be—the DA's office, police training, death investigation, the sheriff's department, lawyer's offices, workman's comp—there are so many places they can work and so few of them are getting jobs.

Getting DAs to accept forensic nurses was difficult at first, but now that they have proven themselves, Arthur Danner III of Santa Cruz Superior Court, who is now a judge, is all for SANEs. One of the best ways to get the DA in your area to come around is to have him talk to other DAs around, who have found that, like the Mounties, "We get our suspects."

Now Sandra and Sherry are on everyone's minds when the DA, FBI, doctors, or other law enforcement groups have questions about sexual assault.

Working in a high-crime area of North Philadelphia, Pat has had a lot of experience with sexual assault. Two friends of her daughter were raped. "I saw first-hand what it did to the family," she says.

One of her first exposures in the ER was a woman who had survived a gang rape. Each member of the gang had initialed her with a Magic Marker. This went to court, and she was able to give evidence that helped put some of them away.

"It's gruesome work at times," Pat says, "and if your focus and your heart isn't in it, you shouldn't be doing it. I spend a lot of my own time giving lectures, giving in-service to the police, labs, women's groups, schools, helping others who want to take the training, not to mention the every-third-Saturday-of-the-month meetings of the Sexual Assault Program, and the DA office, when we have a case."

Because of the work Dr. Ann Burgess has done, rape is now elevated to a legitimate crime. "I'm sure that there are one or two cops who still don't understand what the fuss is about, but no matter where you are, there are always going to be holdouts, people with poor attitudes."

Unlike some of the other SANEs, Pat has the support of her medical director and head nurse. Some of the earlier directors thought that rape was too offensive to deal with and that it was just about hookers not getting paid. But Pat showed them that it happened to middle- and upper-class victims as well. Rape hits close to home, and people often don't want to deal with it. But rape is living forensics.

Still, it's hard for people like the nursing supervisor of Casey's day job to understand why she needs time off for court and for speaking with the DA.

"She doesn't support the SANE program and she puts tons of stipulations on me," Casey says, "like no ER time can be used for SANE cases. This makes it difficult if a case comes in before my shift. That means I am not allowed to clock in until I am finished with *my* case. I lose money and time like that. I'm also not allowed to be on call for SANE while I am on duty in the ER, and that can make coverage difficult."

As one of the Georgia Network to End Sexual Assault (GNESA) nurses, Casey has taken over the training there. Having worked in the ER for over twenty-seven years, she has seen her share of rape, abuse, and violence.

"I hated the way the victims were treated in our ER, but I didn't feel I could do anything more than what I was doing," she says. "I hated the way they were just 'cut loose' to drift through the system. I always dreaded going to court. But several years back I was approached and asked if I would like to train as a SANE.

"There were several other nurses with me; I am the only one of my original group still working. They said the hours and pay stank. It wasn't worth killing themselves for, despite their ideal of justice."

A blurry-eyed Kim fumbled for the phone. It was two a.m.

She'd only just gotten to sleep after her shift at the ER. Having worked a twelve-hour day from seven in the morning to seven at night, and then covering until eleven o'clock because someone called in sick, she was exhausted. Her legs could barely carry her to the car. At home, she had a glass of cold tea. Her head throbbing, she fixed herself a salad, ate, and collapsed.

She had fallen asleep in front of the TV with her cat, Buffy, on her lap.

"Yeah?" she said to the phone.

"We got one for you."

"I'm not on call."

"You're right. Oh, sorry. It's Jane on call," the voice at the other end apologized.

"Oh, all right. I'll come in. I'm already awake."

She arrived at the hospital ER twenty minutes later, having just taken time to pull on a clean uniform and grab some crackers when she realized that she had never finished the salad she'd made.

As the only hospital in a seventy-five-mile radius, Kim's ER took care of absolutely everything in sight.

"God, please don't let this be a bad one," she prayed as she drove back into the hospital parking lot, thinking of the victim she had treated just the night before . . . blood and gore all over the place.

"So, what's going on?" she asked at the desk. The look on the faces of the staff gave her an idea of what she was facing. Shaking their heads, they looked down.

"They're in there," the on-duty nurse said. "I think the cops are talking to her."

When were they going to learn that they all had to work as a team? There were protocols in place. They needed to be followed.

Kim rolled her eyes. It was going to be another one of those nights. She imagined that these cops must be new to the sexual assault unit. Most of the police had been trained by Kim and her colleagues not to start their interview process until the nurse arrived. But some of the new guys—and a few of the old ones— still didn't understand the role of the nurse in the sexual assault exam or of what help she could be to them. They wanted to do it all themselves.

She set down her bag and was immediately approached by the officers, detectives, and media, all wanting to speak with her. Kim knew right away this attack was assumed to be the work of the serial rapist who'd been attacking women on the highway.

"Excuse me," she said, smiling, and pushed her way past the reporters.

Dr. K., the ER attending physician, was already holding court. Kim gave him a half smile. He had been against the SANE program when it first started until he realized how much time and effort it saved him.

It irked her knowing that he would take the credit for discovering the evidence that she would find. He would be the one called to court and paid as an expert witness when he couldn't even describe the injuries properly.

He had already lost one case for Kim by describing the wrong injuries to the court, despite the fact that Kim, when she had done a follow-up as a fact witness, had tried to correct him. The confusion had let the perp get off scot-free. As far as she knew, that hadn't even bothered him.

Yet, like pulling the cart uphill, Kim knew she had to continue trudging or she'd never make any headway in this "game" of the justice system.

Entering the room where the sexual assault victim was being prepared for the exam, Kim greeted the young woman and noted that she had short, brown hair, whereas the other victims of this rapist had been blond. She wondered if that made any difference.

Carefully, she had the victim remove her clothing. One piece at a time was wrapped in clean white sheets and packaged for the crime lab.

She was all business as she took out the forms.

"So tell me again what happened?"

"I already told the police." It was clear the victim was tired, but Kim was, too.

"If I have to go to court on what you are telling me, I need to know as much as I can."

Kim took some photos of what looked like bite marks. If they were, that would fit in with the MO of the rapist whom they had already dubbed the "Highway 10 Rapist," and maybe they could even get some DNA off the area. She swabbed it and air-dried it.

This victim was calmer than the others and able to recall some details of her attacker's features, including the color of the car he drove.

"Three days ago, victim number two also described bushy eyebrows and a blue car," Kim said as an aside to the detective.

"You sure about that?" he asked as he flipped through his notes.

Later, after Kim was finished with the exam and he came back to collect the victim and the evidence, he had to admit that Kim was right.

As she drove home, it seemed to take twice as long as it had going there. Her head ached because she had left her contacts in too long and she was starving.

Pulling into a fast-food place, she took a couple of Advil while she waited for her fish to be ready.

Returning home, she turned off the TV, which she had forgotten before, and, putting on some Indian flute music, she sank into bed.

No sooner had she closed her eyes than the phone rang yet again.

"I'm so sorry, Kim. We have another."

"I'm on my way." She sighed.

It was hard not to think of the times when she had done double backs or overtime and gotten double the pay. For a night like tonight, she would barely gross an extra fifty dollars, almost not enough to put gas in her car for all the trips to and from the hospital!

If only she wasn't so hooked on making a difference in people's lives and in seeing justice done.

It's 5:45 a.m. by the time she finished the second case for the night. At least this hadn't been another Highway 10 victim. "Okay," she said to herself, "my regular shift starts at 6:45—less than an hour from now. Do I want to drive home, put on fresh clothes and makeup, or do I want to find an empty gurney at the hospital and play dead for an hour?"

As usual, Kim opted for the nap and prayed that today would not be a difficult one at the ER.

The staff greeted her with the usual stares. She knew she looked like she'd been run over by a Mack truck. No makeup, hair falling everywhere, clothes rumpled, and bifocals, which they were not used to seeing.

How she made it through the day, she didn't know. She wasn't scheduled to be on call tonight, so she drove through McDonald's and picked up her supper.

She made it home and slid into bed for an extended coma, only to be wakened by the shrill of the phone again.

Sweat pouring over her, she jerked awake. She let the phone ring for a moment before answering, as she got ready for what they were going to say. "Hello."

"Mom, hi, it's me. I just wanted to see how your day was."

Kim didn't even think she should tell her daughter.

No doubt about it, they had to train more people for this, and they had to get the county to pay a decent salary, especially considering all the overtime that the nurses had to go through.

But despite the obstacles she has had to face, she wouldn't give it up for the world. "Knowing that I am making a difference in someone's life, that I am improving the quality of society, makes it all worth it."

In 1976, the first SANE program was developed as a multidisciplinary victim-centered response to sexual assault, among other cases crying for the attention of a trained forensic nurse in the emergency rooms of the country's hospitals.

Like most infants, this program struggled to survive and find its place in society; it had plenty of growing pains, but it did grow. In 1991, when the *Journal of Emergency Nursing* first published its list of SANE programs, it identified only twenty. Today, there are over one hundred and seventeen programs in the United States and Canada. That is still not nearly enough, when you see the statistics that show hundreds of thousands of children and adults raped or assaulted each year and you know what a contribution these SANEs can make to helping victims, identifying the perpetrators, and aiding in their conviction.

The Nurse and the Law

"I remember how as an ER nurse in the early seventies, I once saw the cops come in with a victim and I referred to them in the hippie vernacular as 'pigs.' I didn't really mean it, but I was so used to hearing that and it just came out," said one nurse. "But now we are a team. I can't think of working any cases without them as my partners. Just as nurses, we have, for the most part, better communication skills. That means it is easier for us to talk to the victims and families. We get information that the police would have to work harder at finding. With our assistance, the cops develop their cases quicker and easier. I can get a hold of a chart for them in a few days that they would have to wait six months for as a formal transfer. I can interpret material for them, too, since I understand the medical ramifications. We can win more cases as a team than we could as opponents."

Working with Dr. Ann Burgess in Boston, and on the edge of the new wave of police work, we often consulted with police and they would ask us questions about sexual assault and sexual homicide. We had a good enough relationship with the Boston police. Often the victims asked us to call for them. At times we had to be able to set the scene for them and encourage their sympathies. For example, "You know she's pretty shaken up about what happened tonight. It was pretty bad. I know she's a prostitute but this is not something that anyone, even a prostitute, should have to go through." Because we were sympathetic, the police would be more so. They came to understand that just because a girl is standing on a street corner doesn't mean she wants to be raped, or that just because a girl is scantily clad, it doesn't mean she is giving an open invitation.

We had plenty of interaction with the police and plenty of time to educate them about the aspects of rape. I imagine we had an easier time of it than some of the smaller communities where the nurses didn't have as much contact with the police. The more interaction, the easier it is for the police and nurses to understand each other, to see how they worked, what they needed and where they were coming from. By communicating with the police, we learn what they do and they learn what we do. The respect just naturally follows. We both are working for the same goals, so we need to remember that and work as a team. Not fight one another.

"You can't be defensive with them, I learned," Gail Lenehen says. "Sometimes they will make a comment that I might think sexist or outrageous. I found a way to turn it around by saying something like: 'It sounds like you don't believe her. What do you think is fishy about the story?'

" 'Gail, doesn't it sound strange that she was driven home by the perp?'

" 'On the contrary. We've seen it happen a lot. It's not unheard of for the rapist to be solicitous after the event. Some of the men have the mistaken belief that they are in a "real relationship." They even ask the women if they would like to see them again. If they don't drive them home, they ask them where they want to be dropped off, and they take them there.'

" 'You're kidding!' the cop would respond.

" 'Really,' I'd say. It gave me a good feeling to know that I was educating the cops while also giving credibility to the girl's story.

"I always try to be honest with these guys and tell them exactly what I see and why I think I see it and what else I might look for and why. I will also tell them what the negative findings mean. Sometimes those are almost as important as what we do find.

"I rely on the evidence and facts before me and not the story told me.

"When the cops start to appreciate us and understand that we are here to help them and make their cases stronger, they will help us to work with them as a team.

"I shook my head one evening when they came in with a victim. 'This is a case for *The X-Files*,' I said to them. 'I just can't figure it out.'

" 'Why, what do you mean?' the policemen asked.

" 'Well, there's this inconsistency in her story . . . ' I then told them why I thought there was something fishy in this alleged victim's story. Maybe she'd forgotten something. Or maybe she'd added things. But the point is, I don't automatically side with the supposed victim.

"The most important thing we have to do with our detective associates is to remain credible for them, so that they don't dismiss us as advocates for the victim, so that they don't think we take everything the victim says at face value. I understand that they will often make judgments. Sometimes too quickly. But we have to try and not do the same. We can't attach blame.

"Often I would collaborate with the detectives. One said to me, 'This story doesn't jibe.' He didn't know how to interpret my findings. The victim had been a victim of partially drug-induced amnesia and did not recall all the events leading up to and including her assault. She was remembering just enough facts to throw us off.

"Very diplomatically I said to the patient, 'This is what you said. This is what I have found. Could it have happened this way?'

"The patient was able to recall the elements in a different light—more factual—and we were able to nab the suspect. I think the officer appreciated my nursing communication skills here and the way we work with the victims.

In Tulsa, the sexual assault response team headed by president-elect of IAFN Kathy Bell works directly out of the vice and sex squad of the city police. Theirs is a near-model program.

As a nursing supervisor, Kathy had first been impressed with the medical examiner's office. Death investigation had always fascinated her, but sexual assault investigation has won her over.

Tulsa had an easy transition to this state of affairs. The community had had enough of the violence around them, and, with the media's help, the sexual assault response team was founded.

The city is one of the few places where doctors did not resist the SANEs because they feared they would be losing revenue or that nurses were encroaching on their territory. The timing was right.

The MDs were actually pushing for the SART team to be established. They liked the idea of evading court time and not having to spend the hours necessary for a proper forensic exam. They were pleased to find more available ER beds. Because of the doctors' encouragement, the hospital CEOs were on the nurses' side as well.

What makes it work is that this SART is not owned by just one agency but owes its allegiance to many. The district attorney was a member of the original task force and sat in on the development of it. It was not a case of a single agency ramming it through.

Funding for Tulsa SART came from a variety of sources, including federal government grants. The law offices provided the evidence kits, the hospital provided medications and treatments, while the prosecutor's office covered expert testimony.

Community-based, Tulsa SART does exams at just one hospital but covers the geographic area of five.

Unless the victim needs medical treatment, she does not have to interact with anyone at the hospital directly, except the SANE, the doctor, and the lab. But all the hospital services are available, should they be needed.

It was originally thought that the SART clinic would not even be in the main hospital at all, but in the university setting. But then the idea of security arose. After all, most of the exams were done in the middle of the night, when there was not a lot of staff around.

However, an area with a separate entrance has been found to be the best for the victims, so that they don't have to traipse through the ER to be ogled by everyone. The best SARTs have places where the victim can clean up, where there are fresh clothes to lend her, since her clothing is now evidence and must be packaged away for analysis, and where there are resources for her use.

Kathy has been known to have contact with a victim for as long as several years afterward.

"Of all the cases I see, the majority of the victims of sexual assaults are kids and teens thirteen to fifteen years old," she says. "Most of them have been assaulted by someone they knew . . . it could have been

at a party that got out of hand, it could have been one
of their peers, but usually it is an older person, often a
family friend. Because such behavior takes advantage
of the victim's trust, this is the most damaging blow to
the psyche of the victim."

To Kathy, whose office is in the police department's
sex crimes division, the hardest part of the job is dealing with cases that can't be proved one way or the
other. There may be evidence but not enough to shep-
herd the case through the justice system. She reports
directly to the detective division major, but unofficially
she is part of the mayor's office, on loan to the police.

The first coordinator of the SART team here was not
a nurse, and therefore did not understand the importance of bringing police and nursing science together
in one firm handshake. One advantage of this is the
nurse's ability to translate medicalese. Those reading
and needing the information from the sexual assault reports are not, for the most part, fluent in medical terminology. Kathy cautions her students to write in plain
English. If the police and prosecutors can understand
what is being said, the paperwork doesn't land in
Kathy's office for translation. "It's important for the
officers to see that given this scenario, this and this
type of injury would result.

"It's also important for nurses in the ER and in critical care to recognize evidence and know how to handle it. The more we are familiar with the other side of
our teams (police or nursing), the easier it is for us to
work together. A marriage like this can be made in

heaven, but we all have to work at it for it to succeed, and that means talking to each other."

Victims with questions, or who need further follow-up, also come to Kathy's attention.

Since, in a city the size of Tulsa, Kathy's job as coordinator of the SART does not take up 100 percent of her day, she is able to spend a good part of her hours in community education and outreach. One of her "side jobs" is teaching at the local police academy and in the surrounding areas.

"Everyone here knows what to do with a rape victim and where to go. There is no competition between hospitals, no 'their hospital is getting more patients than ours.'"

Because the study of victimology plays such an important role in finding these rapists, all of the forensic nursing programs have study modules on this, since it is the nurse who often assists the police in putting the pieces of the puzzle together.

Living or dead, those sexually assaulted are still victims. Often in the smaller jurisdictions, the SANEs work along with the homicide detectives and are called in to examine suspected sexual homicides. At times, the nurse will work with her SART agency and other times within the medical examiner's office.

An avid reader of mystery fiction, Sara, a SANE on her first ride-along to a crime scene, had expected to find blood splatters and clues everywhere. Nothing. The victim's studio apartment was spotless. She wondered if the killer had wiped the area clean with something. There was a faintly familiar, almost antiseptic, odor near the body but she could not place it.

The victim's body was damp, as if she had just showered or been washed down. Even her teeth looked polished and clean.

As she assisted with the forensic photographs of the body and scene, Sara noted a prescription bottle in the medicine chest. It was for Tylenol with codeine, ordered by a dentist, Dr. K.

Back at the morgue, Sara prepared to assist the pathologist with the sexual assault exam and autopsy. When he separated the victim's legs, Sara spotted a condom trailing out of the vaginal opening.

The pathologist, not used to sexual assault exams, had nearly discarded it, but Sara caught it and placed it in a separate envelope. She recalled her lectures from the crime lab. They did not want condoms put into the rape kit proper, because often they leaked and contaminated the rest of the kit.

Finding a biohazard bag, Sara gingerly placed the rubber inside and, after sealing it and marking it properly for identification, placed it in the freezer. This would keep the sperm and fluid until the lab could process it.

There wasn't much in the way of trauma to the genital area for evidence-photographing. According to one of the detectives, the condom could have been from a consensual act—not even associated with the murder, but a coincidence. Still, they agreed to follow up on it.

Nearly four weeks later, Sara was allowed to ride along and called in to another crime scene. This time the scene looked more like a fight had taken place. But, to Sara's surprise, the victim had also been showered, her hair washed and combed, like the first victim. The same antiseptic smell was noticeable but only slightly.

"Maybe you're imagining it," one of the detectives said. He didn't smell it.

"Maybe," Sara agreed. And maybe not. She noticed that this victim also had cleanly polished teeth, just like the other victim. She looked in the medicine cabinet wondering if she would find a prescription for Tylenol with codeine, but none was there.

Still, as she assisted with the exam and the autopsy, Sara was not surprised to find a condom falling from the girl's panties. With no biohazard bag handy, she put the dry condom into an empty syringe container, again sealing and labeling it before putting it in the freezer.

After discussing her findings with the detective in charge, Sara discovered that a vial of painkillers had been found in the victim's purse with the same dentist's name on it—and that the dentist himself was already under suspicion.

An attractive man, married, with two children, he should have had no reason to be associated with the women other than that they had been his patients. But his DNA matched up with that in the condoms. Of course, he claimed that he had dated both ladies and his advances had been welcomed . . . but the detectives thought otherwise.

◆ ◆ ◆

When Teddi came into the ER beaten and bruised, Cecilia, the SANE on call, went over the facts with her. The police had taken their report and left to bring the alleged perpetrator, who in this case was Teddi's date, in for questioning.

During the exam, Cecilia noticed a red scratch on Teddi's neck. "Tell me again, what happened? Did his penis enter your vagina or your anus?"

"I don't know," the girl sobbed. "I don't remember. I think so but I'm not sure."

"Okay, I'm going to do an exam of those areas and take some photos for documentation if I see anything. What about this mark below your neck?"

"What mark?" Teddi looked in the mirror. She stared at the red welt for a moment and then said, "Oh, right. He scratched me because I wouldn't spread my legs far enough for him."

"You might want to check under the suspect's nails for possible DNA skin cells from her," Cecilia told the detective.

"But she didn't say anything about being scratched when we were there," the detective said.

"I think the fact probably got lost in her anxiety about the event. That's not unheard of for a victim to forget small facts in her panic to get the whole story out for the police. Later, during the exam, we often hear things that she forgot to mention. Remember, she's had a few minutes to gather her thoughts and she is a bit calmer now than she was when you brought her in."

"Okay," the detective agreed. "We'll check."

Her DNA *was* discovered under his fingernails, just as the nurse had said. A successful prosecution was concluded because the nurse had sat down to talk with the victim, listened carefully, and noticed something that the victim had forgotten about.

Because of inherent discord between hospital-based forensic nurses and doctors who feel threatened by what they perceive as encroachment on their territory, justice frequently becomes a casualty. One director of a SANE program tells this story:

"We were in trial. One of my nurses had done the SANE exam. The attending physician felt that he absolutely had to be there while she was doing the pelvic and sign off on it even though he scarcely looked at the victim. But because he was there, he was called to court—as an expert witness, no less. He didn't want to go. They had to subpoena him.

"When he got to the stand, he incorrectly identified the structures and the injuries.

"Because the doctor was there, they would not let the nurse be an expert witness. But when she got on the stand, she described the injuries correctly, albeit in an area different from the one he did. However, the doctor's word was taken over the nurse's.

"Ultimately, the case was lost, because the defense attorney picked up the fact that the nurse described one area and the doc another. The defense also got the pictures thrown out of court, because the name of the victim wasn't on them.

"In our system, the first picture of every roll has the victim's name. This is a lesson we learned from the DA, so that if one picture is picked out we know that it is this victim's picture. But the doctor hadn't wanted that. So when the defense attorney came to the nurse to ask if this was a photograph of the victim's injury, the nurse could not be sure, as there was no identification on it.

"Since that time, that doctor, who had such a need to be in control and at the bedside, has not come into an exam."

As a sexual assault examiner, I had been practicing for only a short time but I had performed twelve exams. One of my cases, a thirteen-year-old girl who had been assaulted by a family member, was coming to trial. She had several areas of injury and I knew we had a good case.

In my other life as an emergency room nurse, where I had worked for over five years, I was considered knowledgeable about forensics.

To my amazement, when I was called to testify, I realized that the film I had taken of my client had not developed properly. Maybe something was wrong with the camera, maybe something was wrong with the film. I didn't know. All I knew was that nothing came out. I was upset, as you can imagine.

Nevertheless, I was being called as a fact witnesses, to relay what I had seen. Not being qualified as an expert witness, however, I was not allowed to say that this was a pattern of injury from sexual assault and a non-consenting injury that was consistent with rape. As an expert, I could have said that. As a fact witness, what I was allowed to say was limited.

It tore me up that I couldn't tell the jury what was really happening. All I could do was describe this young girl with a bruise on her cervix—a *significant* bruise on her cervix, I might add. That alone is crucial information. But if the jury does not understand why it is so crucial and what it means, then it is hard for them to give the evidence the weight that it deserves.

The DA and my supervisor had worked with me to help me prepare my testimony.

"They're not going to let her testify as an expert," the DA told us.

"Okay," my supervisor said, "then why don't you try and get me in to testify as an expert? At this point, I have done sixty-plus exams. I'm an NP. I can easily qualify as an expert."

The DA grimaced and went into the judge's chambers. He came out a few minutes later, shaking his head. "You're not certified by this state and you're not an MD." Both of us felt sick. "What if you get an MD to testify to this? We can ask . . ."

The DA shook his head. "Judge said it was too late. Said I should have planned this all ahead of time. He said that maybe he will let me call you, if there is time, but don't count on it."

We didn't count on it, but we hoped.

And so we waited and we waited and we waited. We stayed in court the whole day long, waiting.

The jury went out and came back a short time after with an acquittal.

When we asked them why, they told us: "We all thought he was guilty as sin. But we were waiting for your nurse expert to testify about the pattern of the injury and if it was consistent with sexual assault. We kind of guessed that it was, but we needed to hear it."

My supervisor and I glanced at each other helplessly. There was nothing we could do without being given the status as expert witnesses.

In every case I have testified at since, I have gotten a conviction. Most of the time the cases are so overwhelmingly strong that the DA barely has to lift his finger. When we take the evidence properly, there is little for him to do.

So where does our fight for being an expert witness start? With the detectives. Each time a new detective shows up we have to go back to ground level. I have to explain to them that I have done this so many times. If your daughter or granddaughter were attacked, who would you want looking for the evidence? Someone who was a novice or someone who had done the exams over and over? Would you want a surgeon who has done six surgeries or six hundred?

Most of the detectives are grateful that they don't have to stay in the room with me for the full three hours. I tell them I will page them when I am nearing the end.

Working with the DA is a different challenge altogether. Most of them know that their medical knowledge is slim. Usually I have to go over the case with the DA and show him, explain to him, what questions he wants to ask that will bring out the answers he needs to get a conviction. I interpret the medical record not only for information on sexual assault but also on domestic violence.

Neither the detective nor the DA is going to understand the term "posterior injury." As intelligent as they are, we still have to talk plain English to them. They don't understand that our measurements are metric.

In one case I testified on, the victim had anal injury—a three-centimeter tear. The DA did not understand what I was saying. So I translated it into inches . . . and I showed her just how big a tear that would be.

"Oh, that would hurt, wouldn't it?" she said.

I nodded.

Things like this might seem simple to us, because we are used to them, but when we first started out, we didn't know them, either. I might use the medical terminology for the genitalia, and I have to explain to them where that is and what that means. I have to show them how toluene staining helps us, and the significance of bruising on the cervix.

Most people, no matter how intelligent they are,

haven't the foggiest notion of what the human sexual response is, or why a certain bruise will tell us that this is forced sex and not consensual. They don't understand that during normal sex, the cervix and uterus get lifted up and out of the way, by the natural, responding body rhythm, and why these injuries tell me that this was not normal.

The defense attorney asked me: "You indicated that your findings in this case were a bright redness on the cervix. Is that always consistent with trauma? Couldn't it be"—he glanced back at his client and the jury—"some sexually transmitted disease?"

"Are you asking hypothetically or are you referring to this case? If hypothetically, I admit that the redness could be a sign of sexual disease." I paused for effect. "But in this case, there were no other indications of an STD." Luckily, I was prepared, despite the fact that the DA and I had not had time to work through all the possible answers.

The defense attorney stalled and had to change tactics.

A good number of the SANE training programs have classes in courtroom communication but not all. We need to work with the DA and know how to perfect our testimonies. Yes, we can collect the best evidence and identify many injuries, but if we are not prepared properly by the DA for the questions that might be asked, if we can't win in court because we are not prepared, then what good does it do us or the victim?

Because the SANEs come from a wide variety of

backgrounds, not just emergency and not just psychiatry, we can learn from one another. We continue to bring different aspects of our learning to our trainings and to the national conferences held every year, which enables us to think differently about sexual activity and the experiences that our clients are subjected to.

One of the goals of IAFN is to standardize the training, so that there is consistency in the practice of the SANE, so that when we go into court, we can say, "Yes, we always do this, this, and this, because it is protocol." The other goal is to have some appreciation of our work. Once we are certified in the field, we will, we hope, get the credibility we need from the judges who will see the rape collection kit recognized and used properly, who will understand that we nurses, with our advance practice skills, know as much or more than some of the physicians about injury, trauma, and cause of death. As expert witnesses, we will make a difference in people's lives, in court cases, because we will be fighting for the facts and not for any one side.

One of the biggest obstacles in testifying as an expert witness is the standardization of the ways evidence is collected across the state. Depending on where you are, some hospitals or SART units don't even have colposcopes. They are just not funded properly. This is a big disadvantage. If you are at a small hospital and are limited, without grant money, it's a struggle. Where does the future of the SANE/SART program go if criminal justice won't support us?

The collection of evidence and prosecution is, and

should be, a criminal justice response. Any victim can go into Planned Parenthood and get the medications they want to prevent pregnancy and STDs, but they can't get a good forensic exam with evidence collection, and there is no one there to help the victim if she chooses to come forward. Since it is for the police to prove a crime and get the perp off the street, it doesn't make sense that only the hospital should be responsible for the collection of the evidence.

A victim of a violent crime needs to go to a hospital that has forensic capability to collect the evidence, but not all hospitals are equipped for that, because some emergency departments have found such exams too costly to provide. This service really belonged, they decided, with the department of criminal justice.

LEGAL NURSE CONSULTANT

Little Jennifer was born severely deformed, with numerous defects. The family, torn apart by indecision, didn't know what to do. Despite the poor chance of her survival, a heart transplant was ordered by one of the agencies helping the family.

The insurance company did not want to pay for the transplant cost. The nurse in charge of the Medicare claim did not see it as practicable. But the agency persisted.

There were still other problems: Who would pay for the child's ongoing care? Who would help the family survive this terrible situation? What do you do about cases similar to this, where ethics conflicts with the bottom line? The case went before the ethics committee review. As both a legal and medical issue, something like this is a gray area that's difficult to navigate.

Does one do only curative treatment, or palliative, too? Where do the resources come from, and how do you make a decision to use resources for one and not the other, especially when said resources are limited, as state funding always is.

For people caught in the middle, it can be a tough decision. That is why the companies hire forensic nurses to evaluate these cases.

There are several roles for forensic nurses working directly with the legal system.

"Lawyers, doctors, and nurses all speak English, but they don't speak the same English. They think differently," says Deborah, an MSN in oncology who works for the Department of Corporations, Health Division. This department regulates HMOs and other health groups. "We are needed to bridge the gap, jump the synapse between the nursing/medical nerves and the legal nerves. Very often the doctors don't want to speak to the lawyers and the lawyers don't want to speak with the doctors . . . even if they are on the same team."

It's for this reason that so many doctors and nurses go into law to understand what is really going on and to help bridge the gap so they can advise physicians and nurses on legal issues they had not thought about.

(Very few lawyers, it seems, have gone the other route. Most of them are intimidated by medicine.)

As a nurse for the department, Deborah evaluates cases where the patient has a complaint about the health corporation. A cancer survivor herself, Deborah works from her home and can call the patients at hours convenient to her and them. She has enough clinical experience so that the insurance companies can't snow her and say something is not important when she knows it is.

A team of phone staffers takes the initial call to the hotline and writes a concise version of the situation. Most of those working the phone bank don't have any medical knowledge and can only guess if something is important or not.

If it appears urgent, the case is referred to Deborah or one of the other nurses here who will call back and investigate the facts.

"I try to guide them on working through the system, how to file a grievance, how to buy time, without causing distress. But if they have done all they can, or if the issue is life-threatening or serious, as cutting off chemo treatment might be, then I will start making calls myself. My role here is to make sure the urgent needs of the patient are being met."

The cases range from someone not getting preapproval on an experimental drug to use or abuse of treatments, chemo, and the like, to having a contract canceled in the middle of chemo and not knowing how to pay for the rest of the treatments. Most of the time it is the insurance company not wanting to provide something that medically could help the patient—but then it comes down to just how much the patient really will be aided.

The nurses who work here have to be arbitrators and negotiators, bringing two different views to the table.

Deborah pointed out that the patient isn't always right. "Sometimes the patient wants something that is just not appropriate for them or is not what we would consider medically necessary. But when it is, I will call the heads of the HMO personally and force them to give me a response."

"Since we are part of the governor's office, we can get an answer in one to five days. But I don't do medical determinations on quality of care. I prepare a case so that it can go to one of our specialty consultants. All the doctors who work as specialists for us have to be university affiliates with enough credentials so that they can go up against the insurance review boards when they say something is not medically necessary."

Claudia fell into legal nurse consulting. She had been working in the hospital when she was approached by a defense firm needing a bilingual nurse to review Spanish medical records. They had a huge chemical exposure case in Puerto Rico and needed to interpret the medical records. Nineteen claimants and hundreds of medical pages later, she thought it would be a one-time-only event.

This was 1989, when only a few nurses were interpreting medical records and working out chronological timelines so that the lawyers on the case could have quick reference.

Seeing herself as both an advocate for the client and the health care provider, Claudia screens out lawsuits that don't belong in the legal system.

When one does, she gets a proper view of the case and tries to make it worth as much as possible for the client. Her perspective as a nurse helps to maximize the case. Most of her cases are ones where the quality of life is significantly affected for her client. "Once I am committed to a case, I give it my all," she says. "I consult with the best experts, obtaining all the medical records, summarizing and teaching the attorney the medical and nursing aspects of the case, preparing him for deposition and trial.

"Based on the care the patient received, the attorney has to know what to ask. I help him focus on the medical aspect. In preparing the attorney for the deposition, I do all the appropriate research on the medical issues. In a case of septic shock, I do the basic literature search so that they can understand what we are addressing. They should understand what the mechanism of shock is and what it means when the patient is in tachycardia. They should know that blood pressure of 80/50 means the patient is going into shock."

Hiring a nurse to work alongside is one of the best things an attorney can do. An attorney cannot absorb all the medical information or track the information he needs by himself. The nurse reviews the medical records and interprets them for the attorney. She knows where and how to find the documents she needs.

Claudia found several cases where the doctor's orders did not correspond to the nursing notes. (The attorney had missed it completely.) She explained to the attorney what was missing and what it meant.

When the case of a lupus patient who was denied a bone marrow transplant came up in court, Claudia sat in court and wrote down the issues that the attorney needed to address in the cross exam. The answers from the medical experts on the other side were, at times, in medicalese. Despite his knowledge, the attorney could not understand them. Claudia was there to explain it in detail to him and feed him the responses and questions he needed.

"The public needs to know that there is a big difference between the legal nurse consultant (LNC) and the paralegal, who is trained in the legal arts and legal research but most times knows very little about medicine. Head over heels in documents, they don't understand, don't know where to focus their efforts, and they are often glad when an LNC is hired on. There is no way that a paralegal can do what a legal nurse consultant can," Claudia says.

As an LNC, she can serve—and often has served—in the role of expert witness, and as someone who frequently relates to lay people, she can help the jury understand what is happening.

Even if the LNC is not familiar with a particular aspect of medicine, it is easier for her to understand and know exactly what type of experts are needed to comprehend the chart and the case. Sometimes she will subcontract the case out to an expert in pediatrics or psychiatry. Choice of proper experts is crucial.

"Every case I have helped the attorney with, we have gotten a larger settlement," Claudia says.

The case of baby G is an example she offers.

"I've looked at many cases where the baby was not appropriately resuscitated at her delivery, was not properly managed in the newborn nursery, and then was not appropriately transferred to a specialty hospital.

"When baby G was delivered, it was clear from the medical record that something was wrong at birth, but they did not put her on a ventilator. Being a rural hospital, they did not understand the graveness of the situation.

"By the time the transfer team was put together, the baby had suffered hypoxia (lack of oxygen) for over four hours.

"So now I have a baby that has been in fetal distress and is brain-damaged. It wasn't just the OB personnel involved, but the whole hospital, which did not have the proper personnel to get pediatrics involved or an anesthesiologist who could intubate the baby.

"It was a big surprise to the attorney that we had all those people involved. And I showed him what other experts we needed to call upon. The focus of the case totally changed from the birth process to the standard of care given to a newborn and what the newborn nursery consists of in a given hospital.

"I asked the attorney for the intrahospital transfer form.

" 'What?' my attorney asked.

"I explained. The defense attorney claimed no such form existed.

"As a nurse, I knew it had to exist. I asked them to look again. Because, I said, as a nurse, I know that all hospitals do them. And, according to the policy and procedure of this hospital, they do intrahospital transfer forms when sending a patient out.

"The hospital had to testify that they did not do the form, for whatever reason, and that meant they had deviated from their own standard of care.

"I made a point to look at the mother's previous pregnancies and her prenatal history. The attorney hadn't even thought to get the prior records. He didn't know that it was important to check out her previous medical history, and that, since the mother in this case had already had three miscarriages, she was high-risk. The moment she started labor, or even before, she should have been in a specialty setting. Maybe it wouldn't have made a difference, but then maybe it would have.

"My investigations saved not only the plaintiff but the defendant a goodly sum of money. Court cases are expensive these days. Juries are being persuaded that so many of these cases are unfounded and should not be in court. Once we go to court, there is a higher chance of the defendant winning because of that attitude. My job is to weed the ones that don't have a legitimate claim from the ones that do, and help to win the case with the facts and figures before we even go to court."

Although many of the cases LNCs work on are medical malpractice, there are also cases in the criminal courts.

Ramon was accused of attempted murder after pushing a love rival into a storefront grate. The grate had a piece of uneven metal sticking out of it. As Ramon pushed the other man into the fence, he impaled him on that metal, causing his lung to collapse.

"I have been stabbed," the plaintiff stated. "You tried to kill me."

The public defender prompted Ramon to cop a plea.

His family urged him to agree. Only an uncle said, "Why is it attempted murder if he didn't have a weapon?"

The parents and uncle found another attorney, one who would take the case. They had four weeks to prepare. He, in turn, called Claudia.

"I don't know what to do with this," she said. The attorney and the family pleaded with her. Reluctantly, she took the package of medical records, and that is where the case took off.

She read the ER records of the plaintiff, where it indicated that he had been stabbed, so that is where she started . . . with a stab wound expert. She and the stab wound expert she called began to gather evidence and asked for the victim's shirt. In the expert's opinion, the jagged tear they found was not from a stab wound but from a laceration; the metal in question had had a rounded edge and the penetration had been from the force of the fall.

Had Ramon taken the advice of the PD, he would have been in jail. Instead, he made a not-guilty plea and walked out.

Frustrated with the legal system and the way it was interacting with the medical system, Vickie started Certified Legal Nurse Consultants (CLNC).

She made clear that the legal nurse consultant and the nurse trained as a paralegal were not the same. Each uses her nursing skills in the law arena, but in different ways. "Most attorneys do not understand medicalese, and the doctors don't have time to teach them. Detail-oriented, the nurses turn out to be more cost-effective for the attorneys in summarizing medical records. We translate the medical language into something everyone—lawyers, victims, defense, and juries—can understand."

The night baby Parker was delivered prematurely, the heavy snows almost closed the hospital.

The mother, an eighteen-year-old high school senior, had, she said, been careful about her diet, and her alcohol intake had been "almost nothing." Drowsy with the effort of delivery yet anxious about the outcome, she allowed herself to be pushed and prodded into the emergency room.

Everyone was relieved when she made it to the hospital.

It was almost five hours after the mother arrived at the hospital before the baby's head crowned and made its way through the vaginal canal.

From the moment baby Parker made his entrance into the world, it was clear that he was going to have problems. Rather than kicking, crying, and moving his arms, he lay in the delivery nurse's arms, listless. His APGAR score, which measured the baby's immediate health upon delivery, was only 4, but the doctor assured the young woman that her son was just fine.

Out of the mother's earshot, the doctor ordered a neonatal monitoring setup for the baby. He studied her prenatal information. Nothing unusual showed, but then nothing probably would have, since very few tests had been taken. He jotted a note on the nursing record, highly unusual, since he had his own physician's records to write on.

His note, squeezed above that of the nurse who had, on her own, done the monitoring strip, indicated that the baby showed no signs of distress, but that, because of the mother's age, they were doing a monitor anyway.

Apparently seeing that it looked inserted, the doctor asked the nurse to remove the one page and rewrite what she had written but including his notes, squeezing everything in so that all of it still fit on the one page.

It didn't take long for those in the room to realize that baby Parker was severely brain-damaged as a result of lack of oxygen.

If the doctor had ordered the monitor earlier, or if the nurse had been allowed to keep using the one she had started, someone would probably have seen the need to do a C-section. Obedient to the doctor, the nurse did just that.

When the hospital and doctor were sued for malpractice, Vickie began to examine the records.

So where was that strip? Vickie wanted to know. What had happened during the first three hours of the hospitalization and, if the baby was fine during the time, what suddenly went wrong?

It was then she noticed the indentations on the next page, a sure indication to someone trained in forensic document examination, which the legal nurse consultants are, that the document had been recopied.

"We never found those records, but we made the assumption that the baby was in fetal stress from the time they entered the hospital, if not before. The fact that the doctor indicated the test had been done, but no monitor strip could be found, was a dead giveaway that he was covering his ass," Vickie says.

Saturday night, and all the usual crazies were out, including Malcolm, a previously diagnosed paranoid schizophrenic. When his social security money ran out and he could no longer afford his medications and his room at the halfway house, Malcolm began wandering the streets, muttering to himself. That, in and of itself, might have been tolerable to the townspeople, but when a cabbie, not seeing Malcolm's dark clothing on a dark street, nearly ran into him, Malcolm exploded, attacking the cabbie with all the anger he had pent up.

Coming to the aid of the cabbie, four policemen took Malcolm down. Burly and strong as they were, it was almost impossible for them to hold the wiry, angry man.

Brought into the emergency room of the nearest hospital, one not equipped with a psychiatric unit, Malcolm was put into leather restraints.

Not understanding anything, knowing only that some strange man in a yellow car had tried to kill him, Malcolm was furious. He lashed out and screamed, cursing everyone in sight.

The nurses, per doctor's order, gave him an antipsychotic medication. When that didn't calm him, they repeated it and included an anti-anxiety medication as well.

Nothing seemed to touch Malcolm or his anger. Malcolm managed, despite being strapped to the bed, to move the bed into the hall, frightening several of the staff and patients.

The doctor's order had stated that the antipsychotic medication could be repeated every three or four hours, with the anti-anxiety substance in doses of half a cc after two hours. Two hours had not elapsed, but the nurses, not able to reach the doctor for more orders, decided to repeat it again.

After they had moved the bed back into the far corner of the emergency room, they did not check him, as the policy on leather restraints required. They didn't question the fact that he had become very quiet, assuming it was a result of the medication. When someone finally did remember him, he had already expired.

As a legal nurse consultant, AJ was able to instruct the lawyer on what documents he should be receiving at discovery, including the policy and procedure book for the ER.

Looking at the policy and procedure manual, AJ, having worked in trauma himself, was sure that the nurses there had not followed documented procedure, but the treatment of psychotic and dangerous patients in the book he was given disagreed with his thoughts. Then he realized what was wrong.

"These weren't the instructions they were using then," he told the lawyer. He pointed to the dates on the book. "This has been updated since the incident. Tell them you want the original policy and procedure book," he informed the attorney. "You need to get the book that was being used at the time of the event."

"They said they didn't have any copies of that," the secretary told AJ.

"Then they're lying. They are supposed to keep copies of all the policies and protocols on file. Tell them you want it."

The hospital played the waiting game, hemming and hawing, but finally they found the manual dated March 1995, the date of the incident, and AJ was able to show the attorney that the nurses had not even followed their own policy, which was to check people in restraints every fifteen minutes. The procedure had been updated to every thirty minutes in the new book. The attorney had, at first, been dubious about the value of legal

nurse consultants, but when she won her case with the
help that AJ gave her, she knew she had made the right
decision by hiring a nurse consultant.

When John lost his arm in a farming accident, he was
taken to his local hospital. But, unable to treat him, the
doctors decided to airlift the injured man to the nearest
medical center.

A request for preflight intubation (to keep an airway
open) was denied by the doctor. Recognizing a possible airway problem, the nurse had asked for the pre-
caution, just in case something happened en route,
since inserting a tube during flight was difficult. According to Lisa, the LNC (legal nurse consultant) hired
by the attorney, they should not even have taken John
without having the ER doctor intubate him beforehand.

John was restless but appeared stable, the notes said,
when he arrived at the helicopter, but the minute they
closed the doors, he bottomed out.

The family asked an attorney to check it out.

Lisa received the records. "One of the first things I
do is check out the vital signs and lab values," she said.

The rules of flight transfer for a patient indicate that
the patient has to be in stable condition before the
transfer, unless the patient is a burn victim and going to
a burn center.

With a hemoglobin of 4 grams, he was already in
danger. His blood pressure was also low.

In addition, the patient had been on I & O (intake

and output measurement). He had been given intravenous fluid of over nine liters in less than two and a half hours, but no one bothered to chart his output.

With Lisa's help, the attorney was able to prove his case of malpractice.

Nurses can work in insurance firms as well as attorney offices.

Susan described the case of Marti, who had been the victim of an auto accident in a no-fault state. The victim had started exhibiting schizophrenic symptoms, which the family felt were caused by the accident.

"I read the police report and saw that two people had been injured, but their degree of injury, which they were claiming now, was different from what they had said at the time of the accident.

"I realized she needed further evaluation. I had her evaluated by a nationally acknowledged expert. She also found a good rehabilitation person to work with the patient.

"It's a delicate balance between a real problem and a correct resolution. A lot of people think that it's easy, they think they are going to fool the world and not make any effort at recovery. And maybe that is only on a subconscious level. As a nurse, I more easily spotted inconsistency in the neuropsychiatric reports.

"I was able to follow the medical care and see what was legitimate and where there was a lack of work-up and follow-through or a lack of consideration for other differential diagnosis that could be affecting the case.

"Getting her medical reports, I saw that she had a history of a learning disability. The organic brain syndrome might have fired out a few more neurons, and the impaired transmission of the neurological information could cause the psychosis.

"After working on this case, I was nominated by the company to set up a case management program and a task force with the attorney and adjuster to handle the head injury cases."

Susan works not only for the attorney but for the whole insurance company. "My role is broader. I help the claim adjuster make decisions that she used to have to make alone. I can tell them if this case deserves the maximum benefit without going to trial or if the claim is so bogus that there is no case at all. I explain and teach the adjuster how this is so."

Some experts can be very credible and can be bribed by the attorney to say almost anything. Someone who is "just an MD" and does not have forensic training can be put on the stand and made a fool of.

"If he doesn't know how to properly deflect an attack from the other attorney, he will cave in and everyone becomes confused," Susan says.

"As nurses and doctors, we only want people to get better and not have to choose sides. We want to take in all the aspects and various diagnoses that affect this patient, but they have to understand that no deep pocket is really free. Even if you walk away with an extra hundred thousand, your psyche is totally destroyed.

"There is a big difference between a degree in medicine or nursing and understanding the legal perspective of a medical case. In a criminal case, you need to know beyond reasonable doubt. To work as a forensic nurse or physician, you have to understand the legal mind-set, which would rather be antagonistic, since the minute you are in litigation you are on one side or the other.

"So I have to explain medical reality to the attorney. They want to present an appropriate defense, but sometimes the best defense is just to say yes, something serious did happen here. They usually take my advice.

"In a civil case, we only have to prove that what is in question is 50 percent likely, in a criminal case we need much stiffer evidence, but the jury needs to understand all aspects of the case. The knowledge of medicine can help us understand cases quicker and easier than it takes an attorney."

Molly, a seventeen-year-old girl, had eaten in a local fast food restaurant. She claimed to have gotten food poisoning from the hamburger she had there. Based on this, she filed a case.

Her mother gave the attorney Molly's medical records.

Molly claimed to have eaten the food in the early evening, yet the entry stated that she had suffered from stomach pain earlier in the day. It looked like the time of the entry had been changed.

There was also a page missing.

When asked about it, the nurse at the clinic indi-

cated that the mother had called and said that time of
Molly's sickness had been later and could she change
it on the record for her!

In northwest Texas, Marilyn has carved a niche out of legal mediation. When the state takes kids away from their
parents, they expect to terminate the parental rights and
not return the children. Here Marilyn serves as a third,
neutral party. If CPS (Child Protective Services) takes
this to court, there is a court-appointed advocate for the
child, an attorney for the child, and the CPS attorney.
The county and the parents each have their attorneys and
perhaps a case manager for the child. Other possible at-
tendees might be the foster family and any possible
adoptive family. "It's quite a crowd and I am the one
who has to coordinate all the communication," Marilyn
says. "My main concern is what is best for the child."

Marilyn is also part of the state ombudsmen service
where people can take care of their managed care
questions and workman's compensation problems. She
is now helping the doctors to organize a collective bar-
gaining unit and, in addition, works with aviation accidents in helping to reconstruct the scene.

Elana, a legal nurse who works for the office of the
public defender, is a law guardian investigator. Because of her credentials, whenever someone reportedly
abuses kids, Elana is sent out to determine what that
means, what the child is saying versus what the parent
is being accused of doing.

When she finds suspicious indications of abuse, she informs the Department of Social Services, which sends its investigators.

"Many times the children do not want to leave, even when there is abuse. My main job," Elana says, "is to be the voice of the kids. I use nursing assessment skills and check out the children's mental, physical, and scholastic status. The child tells me something and then I assess it myself. If I think it appropriate, I bring it to the attorney for the child. I have gotten clothes for kids, computers for them to use at school, health appointments, and psychiatric evaluations. I will recommend for the child to see a psychiatrist or get treatment for hyperactivity, if needed.

"As a legal nurse consultant, I look to see if there is anything that deviates from the standard of care in a variety of areas, home health, IV therapy, and corrections. I get sent the records, review them, and then I go to court and explain what I found.

"Just as in working with the criminals, with people who you know cannot be rehabilitated, you have to know yourself and be realistic. You have to take the facts as they come and not as they are coated by feelings or the media."

The legal nurse consultant is only as good as her previous experience, or her knowledge of how to find the specialists in the field. Carolyn was one such nurse, who spent a lot of time working in trauma before she started doing legal nurse counseling. "I did a lot of work with the homicide detectives, and I really enjoyed putting the puzzle pieces together. The detectives would understand the ballistics of gun wounds, but not how it translated into why someone would die from that injury, especially as it related to cause and mechanism of death.

"Law enforcement understands one piece, the lawyers understand another, and medicine understands a third. It takes nursing, at the center of the wheel, to pull all the spokes together into a whole. I don't claim to be an expert on anything. No one person can know everything, but I have enough education to pick up the commonality, help them relate to one another, and to glue the pieces together. If they have made a judgment call and I think there is evidence or documentation to the contrary, I'll show them what will present a problem, but I won't threaten their legal ego."

Basically, that's what it's all about, isn't it? All of us working together to solve the puzzles.

Investigating Deaths

A nurse in a forensic nursing program began work on a special study: the rate of premature infant deaths in a particular section of her state. Her original thesis had been that with the coming of the government WIC (food for the Women, Infants, and Children Program) the improved nutritional levels of mothers before birth and of the children after birth would lead to less disease and fewer deaths. But when she began her research, she found a hodgepodge of answers to questions on the death certificates, none of which showed the actual cause, manner or mechanism of death, or condition of the body. In a sample of ten, nine read "cardiac arrest" and one had "respiratory arrest" as the cause of death.

With her knowledge of nursing and medicine, she knew that writing "cardiac arrest" on a death certificate was a cop-out. Leading forensic nurse Virginia

Lynch explains: everyone dies of either a cardiac or respiratory arrest—your heart stops beating and you stop breathing—sometimes one comes first, sometimes the other. They are symptoms of every death; the key is knowing what caused the heart to stop, what caused the lungs to fail, what events led up to that moment in time? And autopsies sometimes don't reveal that secret.

Death certificates without an accurate cause of death are useless. Yet even most doctors and nurses do not know how to fill them out correctly. "Cancer of the lung" could accurately be a cause of death, it starts the chain reaction of events leading to death. When we know that is the cause, it could lead to being able to prevent others from dying in the same way.

A case in point was that of an electrician who had been struck by lightning while repairing an elevator and severely burned. He appeared to be recovering until his wound became infected and he died.

His family wanted his accident insurance to pay for his death, but the company saw that his medical records read that death was due to an infection and was not covered. The employer and the family fought back. Virginia Lynch was brought in as an expert witness and quickly concluded that the case had not been handled properly from the start; it should have been a workman's compensation case. The line of action and reaction was fairly clear cut from the time the lightning hit until the man died, but a health-care worker, not understanding cause and effect, simply listed "infection" as a cause of death. A better certificate would have indicated that the infection was the result of the burns suffered while working during a thunderstorm. Had it been accurately listed as not a natural death, it would have been subject to an investigation by the medical examiner or local coroner.

"Cause of death" could be the injury, the disease, or a combination of the two that is responsible for initiating the events that lead up to the fatal moment. Whereas the "mechanism" is the chemical disturbance or bodily disarrangement that stops life.

Some of the problems arise from this common situation: A nurse complained about her county having no medical examiner. "There is only a coroner. He's elected and all he needs is a pickup truck and people to vote for him."

"When a case of unnatural death comes to court, juries need to know what misinformation can result. They need to know what death investigation system they have in their county and if the person doing the investigation knows anything about medical problems or if he's a hardware store owner who just got elected because he had bucks behind him to buy the election."

When a six-month-old was found lying dead in his crib in a seamy part of town, the nurse-coroner was called in to investigate. Her information reported that the child had no history of disease that would have accounted for his sudden death and there were no reports of abuse by his single mother. The child could have died of SIDS.

The first thing that hit the nurse as she entered the child's room was the odor of vomit. She asked if the baby had been sick and learned that it was his older brother, a three-year-old, who had been ill. He had complained of stomach problems for several days in a row. The mother assumed it had been constipation.

As the nurse-coroner went to examine the body, the steam radiator came on. She saw green paint curling from the pipe that ran through the basement apartment. Her training as a public health nurse alerted her. Lifting the dead baby's lip, she saw the thin bluish "lead" line on his gums and instructed the mom to have her other children tested for lead poisoning at once. She was right; the children all had lead poisoning. A lay coroner would not have looked for this, but the nurse, focused on the signs and symptoms of disease, did. As a former public health nurse, she knew what steps to take to save the lives of the older boy and his sister. Studying the dead can help the living.

There are many values in having a knowledgeable person in the position of death examiner.

When a four-month-old baby girl was put down for her nap, no one suspected that it would be her last. Two hours later her father found her lying still in the crib, not breathing.

Within two minutes of arriving at the emergency room, the baby was pronounced dead. The nurse-deputy

coroner, called in to investigate the sudden death, re-
marked to the nurse there how odd it was that the parents did not insist on coming to the hospital in the
ambulance with their daughter, and had not arrived yet.

The ER nurse defended them; they were upstanding
members of the community. The husband was on the
local church board and the wife was president of the
women's circle. The nurse-coroner shrugged, but she
was not satisfied.

The general decision was that the baby had died of
SIDS (Sudden Infant Death Syndrome). It is a "diagnosis
of exclusion"; if no other cause of death can be found,
SIDS is made the "cause of [a baby's] death." The physician, who knew the father from their country club, wanted
the nurse-coroner to sign a death certificate on the spot.
The nurse, however, wanted to be sure they had checked
every angle before resorting to SIDS, and the doctor had
no choice but to go along, since the nurse was on the
medical examiner's staff as a criminal investigator.

The child had been healthy. Previous medical records
showed no problems, no recent colds. There were no un-
warranted marks on her, nothing that would flag
"abuse." All the autopsy found was some dried blood
near her perineum, the area between the vagina and the
anus. The nurse coroner saw nothing out of order, except
perhaps that the child had a clean fresh diaper on. Usually when a baby awakes from a nap the diapers are wet.

Only several hours later did the parents arrive at the
hospital. The nurse-coroner sat down to interview

them, aware they had just lost their daughter. She assured them that she'd be brief.

The mother, a young woman with huge hollow eyes, sat quietly beside her husband, seemingly willing to let him answer the questions.

"When did you last see her alive? Tell me everything that happened," the nurse asked.

The father's answer was "Nothing." Nothing out of the ordinary had happened. He had put the baby down for her nap. No one else had been in the house at the time; his wife had gone to the store to get him more beer to have while he watched the football game.

The nurse asked if the baby had seemed all right that morning and if she had eaten okay; if she had slept well the night before or had any breathing problems that they had noticed. She asked then what the baby had been dressed in when they put her down for the nap. "We've learned that sometimes children who die of SIDS are dressed too warmly."

Since the baby had a dry diaper on, the nurse-investigator wanted to know who had changed her. They said that the mother had changed the baby before naptime and the dad at halftime, when he had checked her.

When the parents left the doctor said to the nurse-coroner, "You are going to sign it out as SIDS, aren't you?"

The nurse still had a nagging doubt. She said that she would have to come to the house and check out where the baby was napping. Looking at the place of death could tell her a lot.

It was crucial for her to see the scene before it was disturbed. But it was twenty-four hours before the nurse could get permission to check the house. As an attorney, the father said he knew the value of not touching anything and claimed he had not. The paramedics had been instructed to take photos of the scene, but because the community knew the couple, they had not.

Finally, the permission arrived. While a child service worker talked with the parents in the living room, the nurse examined the area where the baby had been sleeping. The crib looked sturdy. Bumper pads protected the side. Everything looked safe, yet something still nagged at the nurse-investigator.

On the floor she saw two crumpled pieces of paper. They were certificates of completion of the examination of a family violence program.

In the crib, she found a body pillow with a stain on it, which was folded over so that the stain was on the inside. She took that for testing, too. Next to it, a broken rocker and an inflatable mattress lay in the baby's room.

There was a crack in the telephone receiver and the wall behind it had a hole.

As she walked into the kitchen, more broken furniture confronted her and another hole in the wall.

The case was looking more and more like infanticide rather than SIDS, but the nurse knew her boss would not let her post that without positive proof.

When the nurse reported back, she told the coroner that she was not ready to sign. She wanted the child death review team.

The multidisciplinary team recorded and transcribed interviews of the family, grandparents, childcare providers, neighbors, and other law enforcement. The medical examiner pointed out that there was no evidence of foul play. He was right. Other than her suspicions, the nurse-investigator had nothing.

Ongoing observation of the parents continued as the nurse-investigator pressed for more time and hoped for something definitive. But as the days stretched into weeks, the chances of finding substance for her suspicions were proving more and more fruitless.

Autopsy on the baby showed nothing that contradicted SIDS. But one of the nurse's key clues was the parents' delay in coming to the emergency room. Her nurse's training in psychosocial aspects of grief counteracted everything she had seen from them. There were other points that bolstered her doubt. The husband was very controlled and it was obvious that his wife was afraid of him. From the papers she had picked up, she knew that the couple had a history of domestic violence.

The investigation dragged on for three months.

Her superiors pressured her continually: "Just sign the baby away as SIDS." She begged for just a few more days.

Finally, she convinced the mother that she could speak without fear. She could get to a shelter where she would be safe. That was the turning point. She finally admitted that her husband had willfully snuffed out their daughter's life.

He was arrested and booked on child abuse, neglect of the infant, and homicide. The behavior of the parents in not accompanying their infant in the ambulance had been what lit the nurse's suspicious fire. Her persistence in investigating the death led to her refusal to be content with diagnosis of SIDS.

One of the first nurse-coroners, Marion C. was elected to the job "probably because no one else wanted it."

She started when she was in the emergency room where a man lay dying, and it was her responsibility to fill in the certificate of death.

Not sure how to proceed, she searched all the manuals and found no written policy telling her what to do when death was imminent. Everything was written in vague legal language and left to interpretation by the elected coroner, who in her state was most often someone with little or no medical knowledge.

When the position came up for reelection, Marion ran for the post, not because she wanted the status but because she saw a need. It was then a part-time job with no salary.

Her competition was another nurse, a retired sheriff, and a chainsaw salesman. At a rally she heard the chain saw salesman say he thought he should win just because he had sold chain saws all over the state. His slogan was "A man for a man's job."

He and the sheriff got only token votes. Marion won over the other nurse.

Marion's first few cases were challenges. A lawyer

representing the family of a dead woman attacked her judgment of suicide. "You are making a criminal of this dead woman," he told her.

Marion replied, "Suicide is a crime. If I compromise on this ruling, which is so obviously a suicide, I will never be able to rule a suicide again." (The lawyer's motive for trying to influence her was self-serving, since the insurance company would pay for an undetermined death, but not for a suicide.)

Slowly she managed to get a small salary and a staff, but it was pulling teeth to make the legislature understand that funds were also needed to take care of victims left behind. "They were a harder tug than a breech baby." Every yard had to be gained painfully in her battle with the county board. Finally they upped the ante to twenty-eight dollars per case and paid her staff a per diem, and she fought for a two-way radio so she'd be safe in the field. Other benefits were nonexistent.

She had hoped to staff her offices with registered nurses. "RNs," she explained, "are ideal for death investigation because their training makes them eager to put pieces of the puzzle together. We can trace the events that lead to the death and show where it began, how it started. That's the only way to learn anything and to prevent further deaths." But so many of her staff were forced to take second jobs to make ends meet that Marion herself ended up with 85 percent of the cases.

The first thing she did when she took office was send a directive to everyone remotely involved in death investigation—police, fire, medical, hospital, paramedics—

so that they would know how to report a death and the
process that she would follow. Because, even though
she was a nurse, she had been in the dark about the process of death investigation for so long, she wanted them
to know step-by-step what was done and what she expected of them and what they could expect of her.

"Here I was, this twenty-six-year-old girl, telling
these cops how to work at a death scene. Some of these
guys were old enough to be my dad. Initially, I received a lot of buff. It was not a good feeling, but then
I proved myself in several cases and after that everything changed."

From her experience as a forensic nurse, she tried to
focus not only on the victims, but on the other players
as well: the police and EMS. She knew that she was not
investigating the crime, but she still could point out
things that were, perhaps because of her education, obvious to her. Sitting and talking with the victim and/or
the survivor's family, she was able to pick up clues.
Nurses focus on communication and work as a bridge
between doctors and their patients, so she could understand what the other professionals, like the police,
wanted. She could ask questions in a softer way and
often get more than the others could. As coroner, she
perceived the need as it developed in front of her eyes.
Each case was unique.

One of her first calls was to a nursing home where
they had never asked for a coroner before. There were
frequent deaths among the aged who lived there, but
they were mostly from natural causes, and the owners

were sure Marian had come to take their license away.
She was pleased—and surprised—that they had called
her. She was asked to check out the body of a Mrs. R.
who had just died.

Since the victim was in her eighties and had a heart
condition, the death could easily have been a natural
one, but Marian didn't want to make any assumptions.

The orderly at the nursing home led her to Mrs. R.'s
room. The shutters had been drawn and the sheet been
pulled over the woman's face. Marion approached the
body ready to start her examination. The orderly was
standing at the door, watching her.

"A nurse will automatically check a patient's vital
signs first," she explained in telling the story. "Not yet
used to the role of coroner, I still did it automatically. I
took hold of Mrs R's frail wrist even though she would
not have a pulse to check. But then I dropped her arm
and quickly picked it up again. Surely I had been mistaken. 'This is Mrs. R?' I asked the orderly.

"He glanced at the chart and confirmed it. 'Expired
12:23 a.m.'

"Well," Marion said, "Mrs. R. is not dead. Her
body's still warm, even if your chart says that she died
almost eight hours ago. I'm still getting a pulse."

He flushed redder than a strawberry in September
and ran for the stethoscope.

Sure enough, the patient had blood pressure . . . a
rather good one at that, despite the fact that she was lying still as a rock. Marion took out her laser penlight
and went over the patient's neurological signs, talking

softly to her all the while, looking for some response. It didn't take long to realize that Mrs. R. had had a stroke. The only thing she could do was to blink her right eye. If Marion hadn't checked her vitals, Mrs. R. could have been carted off to the funeral home, and by then she probably would have been dead, with no one being the wiser!

Prior to Marion's election as coroner, when the police had seen a body, they would call the coroner and leave . . . sometimes several hours before the coroner arrived. Crucial evidence would be lost. Early in her post, Marion instructed the police never to leave a body alone, especially in a suspicious case. A funeral home was never to remove a body from a hospital, nursing home, or any other location without permission from her office. It was a big change for those who were used to doing things on their own.

She began a system of educating the police, firefighters, and funeral directors so that they would know when to call her, how to handle the body, what to touch and what not to touch. Nothing like this had been done in the county before. Now everyone knew the others' roles.

Marion's next stop was the DA's office; here she developed a protocol that stated when the body could be moved and when not. Everything was put in writing, including how the new rules would be reinforced. As a result, Marion's method spread statewide and became standard practice.

As nurse-coroner, Marion's concern was not only

with the dead, but with the living as well. "My philosophy has always been to protect the living through the investigation of death. We need to follow through to make sure that the living are taken care of. The purpose of death investigation is to provide answers so that the living will live better."

Exhausted with the battle for every penny, pleased that her survivor follow-up care program was running as customary and expected, Marion retired as coroner. With the needed backing and the equipment, she might have done more. The hardest part of her job had been finding the resources needed and begging for even her minimal needs, despite giving more than a hundred hours a week to her work.

"It's up to the lawmakers to determine how the public and the survivors will be treated. They do so by what funds they allot to the coroner/medical examiner system."

Canada's Dr. John Butt, formerly of Calgary and now of Nova Scotia, fully agrees with Marion's views, which is why those two provinces almost solely use nurses as death investigators. In fact, in Canada nurses have routinely served as death investigators since the 1970s. Only Ontario, which claims to have enough doctors interested in the field, does not use nurses.

"They can go to the scene and coordinate with the family and follow up with the family and the investigation," said Dr. Graeme Dowling, now Edmonton's chief medical examiner. "Not only can they better communicate with the MDs to find out what disease processes the deceased suffered from, but they can interpret medications and medical records and help the police understand just what is going on here. If they find Cardizam (a heart medication) and there is no other indication of heart disease from their physician, the nurse will know that there is something to check into. Speaking the same language as the doctor, they can understand what is going on and translate it for the police.

"Being the eyes and ears for the medical examiner and forensic pathologist, these nurses who go to the crime/death scenes can better understand the reasons a certain action has happened. The police go to investigate a crime and can make an awful lot of something that is really nothing and vice versa."

Abuse and Neglect

"Abuse" is defined as an act that hurts or injures by maltreatment. There are many sorts—physical abuse, exploitation, sexual abuse, emotional abuse, and/or medical neglect. Victims are primarily people (or animals) that cannot adequately defend themselves from it: children, adolescents, mentally or physically handicapped adults, the aged, or even simply partners, "friends," or lovers. An estimated 10 percent of all children seen in the ER are victims of child abuse. The most serious of their injuries are to the head and abdomen, but abuse is rarely an isolated event. It recurs and recurs, getting progressively worse as the offender isn't stopped.

The magnitude of child abuse is difficult to estimate, because the majority of cases are unreported and unrecognized. The child often cannot or is afraid to talk to others about it, and parents won't, as often they themselves are the perpetrators.

Emergency-room nurses need to develop a high index of suspicion in order to identify abuse and take all means to stop it.

After recording the usual information—sex, past medical history, any problems during pregnancy, recurrent injuries—Geri asked the accompanying adult if there had been any changes in the child's behavior recently. (Changes in a person's behavior almost always signal some physical or emotional change. The girl, Leslie, ten years old, had been brought in because she seemed constantly listless and exhausted, although she had no fever and no other sign of infection.)

"No, not really. Not much."

"Are you the mother?" (It is important to identify the relationship between the caregiver and the child.)

"Oh, yeah. Yeah, I am." The mother seemed to space out. Was she on drugs?

"You're the one that she lives with?"

The mother nodded. "Most of the time. Sometimes she's with her dad. We're divorced."

The nurse wrote it down. "What do you think is wrong?"

Mom shrugged. "Don't know. Maybe drugs."

"What kind of drugs?"

Again a shrug. "She's been awfully clumsy lately. All the time falling."

"I see." Geri glanced at the bruising on the girl's

arms and legs. They were multicolored, in different stages of healing. "Where did you fall, Leslie? What were you doing when you got all your bruises? Were you having fun? Riding a bike or something?" (A history of accident proneness was one of the red flags that keyed an observant nurse into the possibility of abuse.)

The girl shrugged. Like mother, like daughter. "Can you tell me, Mrs. P., if your pregnancy with Leslie was planned?" (Two of the factors that often trigger abuse are a difficult pregnancy or an unplanned one.)

"Huh?"

"Or if you had any difficulties during your pregnancy with her?"

"No, not really. She is kind of a problem sometimes, though. Her school records are . . ." Yet another shrug. "She just drives me crazy sometimes, the way she doesn't pay attention to things."

The nurse nodded. "Why don't I examine Leslie alone?"

"She's my kid. I have a right to be here when you're looking at her." The defensiveness of the mom, plus the vague answers and history of "problems," was enough to make Geri suspicious.

"Please, Mrs. P. It will only be a minute. You can sit outside the door if you want. It's just that there isn't much room to move around in this cubicle and if I am going to examine your daughter properly, I really need to be alone with her."

"Oh, okay."

Alone with the girl, Geri felt more free to question her. "It seems that the injuries you have could have been caused by someone hurting or abusing you. Did anyone hurt you? Are you afraid that someone will?"

Overall the girl showed normal development. But Geri knew that her turtleneck sweater—the day was very hot—could be a sign that she wanted to hide sores and injuries. "Can you take off your sweater?"

"I'd rather not." That was further telling. Of course there were cultural and religious considerations that might be holding the girl back, but Geri had not been aware of anything like that in the history. "I really would like to check you out and see if we can come up with a reason for your listlessness. Has anyone hurt you?"

Slowly, a slight nod came.

"And that's how you got all those bruises?"

There was silence a moment. "You're not going to tell Mom that I said anything, are you?"

Geri couldn't lie to the girl. "Actually, if I think there is reason to make a report to the authorities, then I have to do it." She explained to the girl about nurses being mandated reporters of crime. "But if you trust me and tell me what happened, I will do my best to help you get out of a bad situation and protect you. I can't promise you anything but that I will do my best."

"Oh. I love my mom." Words that should have been said with passion were dull and flat, as if the girl thought she was supposed to say that.

"I'm sure you do." Even kids who had the worst history of abuse loved the parent whom they had bonded with, because that was whom they saw as providing for their needs, sporadic as it might be. Abuse victims of every kind were quick to defend the abuser, because they had joined the offender who accused them of being at fault and the cause of the abuse they suffered.

"Your mother says she thinks you've used drugs. Can you tell me about that?"

Leslie shook her head. "I haven't. Well, maybe I tried a joint when my brother had some. But not really. I didn't like it."

"How many times?"

She shrugged. "Not many. Just once or twice."

"So then what's going on?"

"It's my brother," Leslie said after a longer silence. "He hits me and kicks me and pinches me. He says he's going to kill me."

"How old is your brother?"

"Fifteen. *He* uses drugs. I saw him. More than once. I don't think Mom knows, though. I tried to tell her but she wouldn't listen."

"Does she know that your brother does these things to you?"

"He tells her that I fell. Usually it's when he's taking care of me."

"Does she believe him?"

Tears welled up in the young girl's eyes. She nodded. "She doesn't want to believe any different."

During the rest of the conversation, Geri also found out that the brother had sexually abused the young girl. As per protocol, Geri did a sexual assault exam. When the evidence indicated that something untoward had transpired, she collected it, took photos with the colposcope, and sealed it all with evidence tape. As soon as the police arrived, she would turn it over to them and only to them, after they had signed it off. This step was necessary to maintain the chain of custody and make sure that the evidence was useable in court, should the need for that arise. Then she documented what she saw using a body map, photos, and notes.

"Are you willing to talk to the police?"

"Will they take my brother away?"

"I can't answer that, honey. All I can say is that there probably will be an investigation. You might get sent to a foster home until they figure out what exactly is going on. Most likely, your brother will be asked to get some kind of treatment."

"And then everything will be all right again?"

Geri put her arm around the ten-year-old. "I wish I could say it would be, but I don't know. All I know is that until we get you out of this situation, things will keep getting worse. Leslie, no one has a right to treat you like you just described your brother doing. No one has a right to abuse you. I want you to remember that and I want you to talk to someone about your feelings so that you can recover from this."

The girl shrugged. "Okay. I'll talk to the police."

As Geri predicted, the investigation showed the brother to be sexually and physically abusing his younger sister. He was sentenced to a group home, and Leslie went to a foster home. Geri didn't know if that would do anything to improve his attitude or his abuse, but at least he was out of the house and Leslie could return. The mother never fully accepted the fact that her son, her darling boy, had been an abuser. She made life so difficult for the girl that in the end, Leslie moved back in with her foster parents, where she remains to this day. Her brother is still in a treatment facility.

Many of the symptoms of abuse can be the same as those of a different situation, one that is devoid of any wrongdoing. We can too quickly jump to the wrong conclusion. Like the witch hunters of Salem, we sometimes identify as sexual abuse many things that are not.

The nurses in charge of an overnight camp for young girls noticed some blood spots on the underwear of a six-year-old girl. They suspected sexual abuse and questioned the girl.

"Yes, my daddy touched me. He always gives me baths," she said.

Believing they had confirmation, the law arrested the father.

A forensic nurse was asked to examine the girl. She found a normal hymen, no tags or tears, and no detectable anal lesions. Because the girl had complained of pain when she urinated, the nurse took a urinalysis. White cells, or leukocytes, indicated infection, and red blood cells were also noted, accounting for the blood drops on the girl's underwear.

An antibiotic treatment cured the urinary tract infection, and the symptoms cleared up.

The innocent father was released, but his reputation remained sadly besmirched.

There are times, however, when the complaint is valid but there are no symptoms. Peter, a seven-year-old boy, came to the ER with his mother. She said that he claimed he had been assaulted twenty-four hours before by his stepmother's sixty-six-year-old father.

"Is there anything that might cause you to believe what he's saying?" the nurse asked the boy's mother.

The mother shook her head. "But he usually doesn't lie to me."

Often kids are brought to the ER with a wide variety of complaints, like abdominal pains or headaches—pains for which there is no identifiable cause. Peter's mother had not even been suspicious of anything until her son had told her.

"Can you tell me what happened?" the nurse asked. "Are you bleeding someplace? Does something hurt?"

"No."

"Did you hurt before and it went away now?"

"I don't think so."

Not having been trained as a sexual assault examiner, the emergency room nurse was doubtful that anything had happened. After all, she had always thought that rape meant force. Force to her meant that there would be bleeding and pain.

Nevertheless, the boy and his parents continued to insist that a full exam be done, and so the ER nurse called in Kathy, the SANE on call. It was just as well. Because it is often easier for the child to talk to the nurse alone, Peter was brought into an interview room, away from the frenetic activity of the emergency room. His mother was asked to wait outside. Most parents want to be with their child when he or she is being interviewed, but it is not a good idea for many reasons, not the least of which is that they might know the offender and either not believe their son, or cause the son to doubt his own judgment. Especially when it is a family friend, the child could have feelings of divided loyalty.

Parents need to understand that it is in the best interests of the child to talk to the staff alone even if the offender is not the parent. Even if the parents stay in the room but remain silent, the child will sense their anxiety and won't be willing to talk. They often misinterpret their parents' distress as anger directed toward them for wrongdoing.

Having a healthy level of suspicion, the SANE followed the protocol carefully when she did the exam. First she had to determine whether the suspicions of sexual abuse could be confirmed. Since the offenders were so often family members, it was important for the nurse to determine if it was safe for the boy to return home or whether the child would face further victimization. She also wanted to make arrangements for psychiatric follow-up to deal with the psychological trauma of the assault.

While the SANE was examining the boy, another staff member had taken the parents aside to talk with them and find out what they knew and what they suspected.

First the nurse examined the perianal region, between the penis and anus. Both this and the muscles surrounding the anus, or the anal sphincter, seemed normal. If rape is suspected, there could be signs of forced entry, but, as the SANE knew, the absence of injury might simply mean the victim was too frightened to resist, the fright itself being a large part of the resulting trauma. Rarely is physical force necessary with these children. The other possibility was that the assailant had used a lubricant to grease the anal sphincter, which would prevent at least some and possibly all injury.

The proctoscope showed no evidence of trauma to the anal canal. Despite that, the SANE took the boy's word and, just in case, took a swab of the area. Tests detected sperm. DNA proved conclusively the identity of the assailant, who was quickly arrested.

The boy drew a picture of himself showing a prominent mouth and genitals, indicating his increased awareness of them after being sexually victimized. His outstretched arms showed how helpless and vulnerable he felt.

"I didn't want to believe him," his mother said. She was glad that the boy had insisted on the exam but she feared how it would now affect him. "Is he going to be queer?" she asked.

Male victims are often unreported, because the abuse usually involves a male offender. It is often wrongly seen as a threat to the young male's masculinity. If it is reported, they feel that the boy will be labeled homosexual.

Low self-esteem and feelings of guilt are the terrible consequences of so many of these episodes. Whether or not the child appears to have consented, it is still abuse—obviously, the child is not old enough to give permission. Often children are intimidated or coerced into action by means of promises, bribes, or threats. They are made to believe that they are at fault for what has happened and that they will be sent away from their parents if they tell.

In three-year-old Marla's case, she was warned by the offender that if she told she would go to foster care for the rest of her life and never see her folks again, that they would be put in jail and it would be her fault.

Using anatomically correct dolls, the SANE first identified the names that Marla used for her private parts. Most kids do not know the terms "penis" and "vagina" but refer to them as "wee-wee" or "pooh-pee."

In a room that was designed for children, with colorful posters, dolls, drawing pads and crayons, and small tables, Kathy began to talk to Marla. Her first step was to establish rapport, trust, and credibility with the victim. Using short sentences and straightforward talk, Kathy sat down at one of the miniature tables with the little Marla.

"I'm Kathy. I work here in the hospital. One of my jobs is to talk to young ladies like you. I help children who have had bad things happen to them."

"Really? Honest?"

"Honest." Kathy held up her hand.

"This happened to other kids?"

Kathy nodded.

It is important to let the child know that he or she is not alone, that other children have suffered the same sort of thing. Children, like adults, often feel alone in their situation and need to know that others have had the same traumatic experience.

"Tell me, do you like Barney?" Kathy referred to the TV's purple dinosaur popular with most children.

Marla nodded. "BJ's my favorite." He was the dinosaur's yellow sidekick.

"What else do you watch?"

"*Comfy Couch*. Uh, *Rugrats*."

"I like those, too," Kathy said. "I sometimes watch them with my daughter. Do you have any pets? We have a dog named Patches."

The girl nodded. "Waldo is my puppy. He's a cocker."

"How very nice. Marla, do you know why you're here?"

"Mommy said we had to come."

"I want to talk with you about what happened to you. Do you have any questions?"

"Are you going to tell Mommy?"

"How do you feel about that?"

"I don't want you to. She'll be mad at me. I don't want you to," the child said again.

"I think she's upset, Marla, but not at you. She's upset at the person who did this to you."

"Not at me?"

Kathy shook her head. "No, not at you."

"Still, don't tell her," Marla mumbled, and looked down.

"I can't promise that, honey. I have to tell your mom and some other people so we can help other kids like you. You do want to help other kids like you, don't you?"

Marla shrugged. "Guess so."

"I bet Barney and BJ would help other kids."

Marla nodded. "Okay." She gave a big sigh.

Once she had begun to tell the story of her mom's boyfriend, Alan, taking her to the movies and the park, the nurse let her talk.

Kathy was careful not to interrupt the flow of the story with questions, because she knew it might be difficult to get the child back on the same track again. She also knew that she had to watch that she didn't show any negative feelings. Questions like "Who hurt you?" had to be avoided. Most children understand hurt as a physical pain. The child may not have been physically hurt by the sexual abuse.

Very often the offender has slowly built up to the point that he wanted to reach by very tiny advances. It is important to determine exactly what happened. Questions such as "Did anyone ever touch you in some way you didn't like?" help to get the story out of the child, especially one who is reluctant to talk.

"Did anyone ever ask you if they could touch you in a private place?"

"Did anyone ever make you take your clothes off when you didn't want to?"

"Has any grown-up ever asked you to keep a secret?"

Questions like "Who did this bad, bad thing to you?" will intensify the child's anxiety, especially if the interviewer also has negative facial expressions and body language. Even young kids know when they are upsetting someone. Often they will blame themselves.

Marla had to get a clear feeling that nothing she did was wrong, but that the offender was wrong. "Grown-ups are not supposed to do things like that to children."

If the offender has already been identified, it may be easier to get the child to talk. If no person has been mentioned, then the parents need to think of who had access to the child—older kids, adolescents, babysitters, day-care teachers, scout leaders, relatives, neighbors. Stepdads and boyfriends account for a large number of offenders, since they usually have the best access to the kids, but, of course, this is not always the case.

Even though most offenders are male adults, females need to be kept in mind, too, since women have been known to sexually abuse kids.

In drawing a picture of herself, Marla showed her eyes, nose, mouth, and then a huge area for her "weewee." This is where Alan had touched her, she said.

There are several different types of sexual activity that an offender can inflict on a child. He can:

- exhibit himself and look at the child
- fondle the genitals, breasts, and buttocks
- penetrate the vagina or rectum with his finger
- touch them with his mouth
- touch the genitals with his penis
- have actual vaginal intercourse
- have actual rectal intercourse
- take photos of the child in various poses

Kathy wanted to find out when and how often the contact took place. Since most children do not remember dates, Kathy gave her possible events. It was important to be able to verify whether the offender really had access to the child then. "Did this happen before Christmas or after? Did it happen near your birthday?"

Since in this case it had happened only once, Marla was able to recall the time more specifically. Most sexual abuse is repeated and occurs over an extended period of time.

Kathy wanted to find out what kind of coercion Alan had used. "Did he tell you to keep this a secret?"

"He said we were playing a game. But I didn't like it. I didn't want to play the game. He got mad at me and said he wouldn't love me anymore."

For medico-legal purposes, Kathy needed to know if there had been any penetration. This, however, is difficult for most kids to understand. "Can you show me on the [anatomically correct] dolls what Alan did?"

Because of child porn, another question asked is "Did Alan take any pictures of you? What were you wearing or doing when he took the pictures?"

Kathy's interview with Marla was the key in helping to get the offender off the streets. She provided a supportive, nontraumatic environment for the child to talk about the events and her feelings.

A case that was originally misunderstood was a lesson for the nurse: before labeling a particular situation "child abuse," it is important to take into account the culture of the family involved.

Lin, a young Vietnamese boy, was brought in with complaints of a bellyache.

Doing the exam, we found several small, recently made, circular burns on his back.

Suspecting child abuse but not quite sure just what had happened, the nurse practitioner ordered a free air study, which showed that the pains were probably due to constipation.

The parents were unable to explain the burns on his back, but as we took a history for our report, the mother revealed that she had the same type of burns on her own back. She told us that she had recently had a bad cold and explained the Vietnamese practice of "coining," in which coins are heated and placed on the skin to "pull out the sickness."

Had we not investigated, we could have had a false

report of child abuse. While we, of course, did not agree with the practice, we hesitated to report it to Children and Family Services, but we did explain to the woman that hot coins could do nothing for the cold. They could only burn the skin, and that while she might have been following a practice accepted in her country, it was not accepted in ours.

Elder abuse rates almost as high as child abuse in today's emergency room, though it is noticed even less. While very young children often can't talk or can't formulate what has happened, elderly adults, afraid that a complaint about treatment will land them in a nursing home, will refuse to talk. Fear of institutionalization outweighs their fear of abuse or neglect.

As a society we have recently started addressing other kinds of abuse—battered women, child abuse—but we haven't done much for the elderly.

In 1900, only one in twenty-five Americans were over sixty-five years of age. Today, it is one in nine, with the group of over eighty growing yearly. The result is that not only the health-care systems but the family-care providers are overloaded. With older people beginning to become a more significant percent of the population, they will more frequently become our forensic cases.

In 1980, Massachusetts law defined abuse as any physical contact that harms or is likely to harm another person.

Neglect is defined as failure to provide treatment

and services necessary to maintain the health and safety of the person.

Mistreatment is defined as the use of medications, isolation, or of physical or chemical restraint that harms or is likely to harm the person.

Although their cases are similar to those of the victims of domestic violence, elderly victims have special characteristics that make them more vulnerable to the abuse. They may arrive at the hospital on their own, but the story they'll tell will not fit the pattern of injury, and the nurse will need to be a detective to puzzle out the circumstances. And even when it is determined that abuse has occurred, there are very few services to help the victims.

Elderly individuals who show injuries such as bruising around the face, upper arms, or chest are likely abuse victims.

When Mrs. M. arrived in the emergency room by ambulance, the staff noted that her right eye was swelling; it looked as if it had been hit. Each arm showed bruises in roughly the same place, as if she had been grabbed there and shaken. She was confused and combative, and her blood tests indicated that she was dehydrated.

Since the injuries were healing, Janet, the nurse on staff, took pictures of them so that there would be a record for the chart. (There is a gray area of consent here. Mrs. M. was unable to give consent for the photos. Her son, whom they suspected of causing the bruises, would most likely not give it. Janet felt that Mrs. M.'s problem might become a legal case, and, as someone forensically aware, knew that there would be no case, or at best a much weaker one, if pictures were not taken. So she called the district attorney and obtained a court order to take the photos.)

Two days later, Mrs. M.'s confusion had cleared. She was able to discuss what had happened. Having owned her own house for many years, she was no longer able to keep it up. Her son, Jackie, who was mildly retarded, visited her daily. Although he wasn't able to hold down a job, he managed to take care of himself, and lived a few blocks from his mother in a state-run boardinghouse.

His major problem was impulse control, which was poor, especially when he was frightened. At these times, he resorted to physical assault. His mother's aging and decline frustrated him, since she could not care either for herself or for him, as she had in her younger years. He would tell her she had to try harder, and strike her when she did not.

Janet, the nurse, was at a loss in this case. She wanted Mrs. M. to file a restraining order against her son.

Mrs. M. adamantly refused. "Leave him alone," she told the staff.

Since state laws gave the elderly rights of self-determination, the nurse and staff of the ER could do nothing unless they proved Mrs. M. mentally incompetent.

"Okay. What if we bring in a homemaker on a daily

basis to help you?" she suggested to the woman. "If she finds any more bruises on you, will you let us make a report and get a restraining order? I took photographs of your injuries and they're in the chart in case you need them for the court order," she told the older woman. The nurse explained that nothing could be done with the photos without her consent, unless it was decided to file a criminal case if something further happened to her, which she sincerely hoped would not.

Reluctantly, Mrs. M. agreed.

As it turned out, Jackie acted like a gentleman in the presence of the third person, the homemaker. Temporarily, the situation was resolved. Had the forensic nurse not acted with a preemptive strike, and Mrs. M. had returned home to the same problem, it could have resulted in her death.

We seem to tolerate neglect and abuse of the elderly more than we do abuse of children.

Mr. S., eighty years old, came to his doctor's office regularly with various odd aches and pains. While the doctor saw several bruises, Mr. S. said they were a result of falls or of hitting furniture when he stumbled. The doctor was willing to believe whatever the patient said. His nurse, Sammie, wasn't. She was informed about forensic nursing, and questioned him further. The second time he came in with a broken wrist, Sammie sat down with him.

"Would you like me to arrange for a social worker to come over?"

"Whatever for?" Mr. S. responded angrily. "You don't believe me. That's it." He stood, righteously indignant. "What's the matter with my word? You think I'd lie about falling? You think I like having these black-and-blue marks?"

"I'm sure you don't, Mr. S. Do you live alone?"

The old man's facade crumbled. He sank into the chair near her desk. "No. My daughter lives with me."

"And how is your relationship with her?"

"You really want to know?"

The nurse noticed that Mr. S.'s hand trembled now. "Yes, I really want to know."

The old man took a deep breath and sighed. "Not so great."

"How not so great?"

He shrugged. "Just not so great."

"Is it financial?"

Tears were in his eyes. "No. Not really. I have money. That's not a problem. I let Shirley, my daughter, buy whatever she wants for the house, for herself, and for her son." There was a long silence. "I guess I wasn't such a great dad when Shirley was growing up."

"Can you tell me what you mean? In what way were you 'not a great dad'?"

Another shrug. His voice trembled as the waves of emotion washed over him. "She says that I hit her. A lot. That I was abusive. That it was my fault her mother killed herself with drink. She says . . ." The tears poured out now. "I don't remember any of it. Honestly, I don't. I did the best I could to raise her. I remember us walking hand in hand in the park." He wiped his eyes with the tissue that Sammie handed him. "She says I threw hot coffee on her that day when we were in the park because I was angry at something she said. But I didn't," he said, using the denial that most abusers use to block out memories of their violence. "At least I don't recall it." He shook his head, lost in a fog of memory.

"And tell me, Mr. S., what's happening now?"

"Please, some water."

The nurse handed him a paper cup.

As he reached for the cup, she saw round sores on his hand, which might have been made by cigarette burns.

"I understand that this is hard for you to talk about and that you don't recall it, but you must believe that there is some validity to what she says if you are accepting it."

"I was very upset when my wife died. I remember crying at her funeral. That was the first time my daughter and my son said something to me about my being responsible for her death. But she died of natural causes."

"Is it possible that her spirit died before that? Maybe she died because she no longer had the will to live."

He was still crying. "I gave her everything. A nice home. Cars. Even a fur coat. She never understood me. And I guess I never understood her."

"Did you ever physically abuse your wife?"

Mr. S. hung his head. "I seem to recall I might have punched her once or twice. But nothing really bad. They were just love taps. And it was usually for her own good. I am just as sure that if the coffee incident occurred, my Shirley must have done something that upset me. Maybe she was going to do something that would have hurt herself?"

"Well, not having been there, I can't make any judgment about your past, but it sounds like you feel guilty for the way you treated your family. Maybe we should see if we can get you into Riverside Home," the nurse said, referring to a retirement home in their community. "You can have your own apartment there and—"

"I'm not going into any damned nursing home. That's what Shirley threatened would happen if I told anyone." His good fist clenched. "I was born in this house and I am going to die in this house."

Sammie felt at a loss. Clearly she could not let the daughter continue with her abuse of the father, no matter how justified Shirley felt. Yet the patient, being of sound mind and body, had to be the one who made the decision. "Do you think it would help if I talked with her? Or if I had someone from social services talk with her?"

"No. No, you can't."

"Mr. S., if you have money, as you said, why don't you set up your daughter in another apartment? If you don't want to move, maybe we can get someone to care for you. I don't think that living with your daughter is a good idea right now."

"You won't tell the police about what I said. Shirley said they would throw me into a home if I told them."

"We nurses are mandated to report violence when we see it, but I can't make you talk to the police, and if you don't file a report, they can't do anything unless the DA decides that there is a case. He probably won't if you get someone else to take care of you and get Shirley out of there."

As it turned out, Mr. S. did go into Riverside Home, an independent retirement community where he had his own apartment but could have assistance when he needed it. No report was filed against his daughter, who continued to live in the family home.

Marianna, a home health nurse who also had a part-time job with a SART team, used to enjoy visiting Rhoda. The visits were a pleasure. From years of hard work and saving, Rhoda was comfortably well off, living in a nicer part of the city. She had also been left a good settlement from her husband's estate.

The old lady's cardiac condition had been stable, and so had her diabetes, but in the past few visits Marianna made, Rhoda had been irritable.

"What's your sugar level been, Rhoda?"

"I don't know. My son's been taking it. Here." She handed the nurse her book with the times and dates of tests.

Marianna stared at the book. She couldn't believe what she was reading. Sugar levels way above normal . . . in the 200s mostly, but a few higher.

"Are you taking the same amount of insulin?"

"Sure. Same as always. I can't see as well now. So Dave, my son, is giving me the injections."

"I see." The nurse didn't see. If Rhoda was really receiving that much regular and NPH (long-acting) insulin, she shouldn't be having sugar levels this high.

"Okay, let's check your legs." One of Rhoda's problems had been swelling of her legs. Usually they weren't that bad, and if the old woman watched her salt intake, she had no trouble with them. But this time, Marianna asked, "What have you been eating, Rhoda?" The legs were like two pink sausages packed tight. Water glistened on the skin. That meant they were weeping, not a good sign.

"Yeah, they've been bothering me a bit."

"But what have you been eating?"

The older woman shrugged. "I don't know. Since Dave moved in to take care of me, I've been letting him do the cooking."

"He knows you're on a low-salt diet?"

Rhoda nodded. "I gave him all the stuff you handed me."

Then Marianna noted the black-and-blue marks on Rhoda's inner thighs.

"What's that from? Did you go bike riding?" the nurse asked, trying to make light of the situation.

"What?" The older lady looked down. "Oh. Nothing."

It looked like finger-pressure marks, but Marianna couldn't be sure. However, having the suspicious mind of a forensic nurse, Mariana already had her thoughts of what it might be.

Aware of the forensic implications of what she was doing, she asked, "Might I take some photos of these? I'd like to show them to your doctor."

Rhoda hesitated. She looked away, toward a picture of her family in what must have been nicer times.

"Go ahead." The voice seemed far away.

As it turned out, Rhoda's son, Dave, anxious for her to die so that he could inherit her small fortune for his sagging business, had purposely ignored her health requirements and had at times abused her. But she had been loath to say anything at all for fear of her future and fear of what would happen to him. Rhoda felt sure that it was her fault in the way she raised her boy that made him act the way he was doing now, and she did not want him to suffer for her being "an inadequate mother."

She was relieved when the nurse started the process, which did include a restraining order. Rhoda's will was changed, and an annuity was set up for her son's children so that she did not feel guilty about their future if her son's business did not do well.

As forensic nurses, we have sought to become more careful in the questioning of our elderly clients. We do not just take physical and mental decline as an inevitable part of aging, but, with our more suspicious minds, we think of the other possibilities—of poor care and neglect or abuse. And, unfortunately, we sometimes find them.

Till Death Do Us Part?

Until recently, no one really concerned themselves much with domestic violence. But Nicole Simpson's death and the subsequent O. J. Simpson trial further increased awareness of the situation affecting so many women.

Like a cancer growing steadily, domestic violence is proliferating. The numbers tell us that every twelve seconds a woman is beaten by her husband or partner. Studies show that up to half of all women are physically abused by their partners, and every eighteen days at least one woman is killed by her partner. The abuse crosses all physical, cultural, and socioeconomic lines. Up to 80 percent of suicides and suicidal attempts by women are a direct result of domestic violence. Children who witness the abuse heaped on their parent often become abusers themselves, or get involved in abusive relationships.

The issue of power and control is always at the center of this abuse.

Judy had been on and off medications for depression when she took her infant daughter to a friend's house, closed and locked her house door, and turned on the gas. At thirty-five, she was tired of the arguments, of the blaming, and of her life. Her husband was rich. He could easily provide for their infant daughter. She was just not needed.

Luckily for her, Kara, her daughter from a previous marriage, came home that day early from school with a stomachache. She pounded on the door, wondering why her key did not work. Going around to the kitchen door, which was usually unlocked, she smelled the gas.

"Mother!" Kara pounded on the door. "Mother!"

There was no answer from inside.

She knew her mother had been unhappy lately. She knew her stepdad had been screaming that he wanted a divorce, but she had not expected this.

Calling 911, she helped the paramedics break into the house. Judy lay in front of the stove, unconscious. Beside her was a note: "I can't take this life anymore. Please take care of the baby. Love, Mom."

She was rushed to the hospital, where the ER nurse immediately recognized Judy as someone whom she had just sent home a few days ago.

When she had recovered enough, Judy was interviewed by Pat, a nurse practitioner with a degree in psychology and skills as a forensic nurse. "Are you afraid of anything? Or has anyone hurt you?" Pat asked

Judy. She knew that Judy had a long history of falls, trips, and accidents . . . but until now no one had put them together. She had already figured out the puzzle, but she needed the patient to verbalize the picture.

It took a few minutes for Judy to answer, but finally she nodded.

"Do you want to talk about it?" Pat asked.

Judy shook her head and closed her eyes.

Pat noted in the record that there were bruises of various ages on her arms, where they would be hidden by her long sleeves.

Despite being unwilling to talk about her bruises, the patient allowed Pat to do a forensic exam and take photos of the injuries. This later helped Judy to establish her claim of domestic abuse and helped her to keep her infant daughter, since the husband wanted to fight for custody because his wife was "crazy."

As soon as she was stabilized, Judy was admitted to the psychiatric ward.

She refused to see her husband or her family for nearly four days.

Pat, the forensic nurse who had taken care of the patient in the emergency room, followed up with her on the ward.

The first day Judy could only cry. It took two more days of visits and sitting quietly with the nurse before Judy was able to open up and talk of her fears.

Judy's self-esteem was zilch. Her husband had successfully pummeled any life out of his wife. Her spirit had been crushed like grapes in the juice presser.

Judy's family were Armenian. She was ashamed that others outside of their tight-knit community would see and know of the problem. She was told she would bring shame to her husband's family and his name. Even her own parents were against her leaving him.

"He's a good man," they told her. "He takes care of you and Kara, too. Don't complain so much. It is a woman's place to listen to her husband and to follow his lead."

Pat wasn't surprised. Domestic violence spanned all cultures, religions, lifestyles, and socioeconomic strata. Many of the groups had their own internal way of dealing with abuse, but most just looked the other way and waited for it to go away. They hoped that if they did not make an announcement of it to the world, no one would notice. This made the situation more difficult for the survivors. It made them question themselves, "Why me? What did I do wrong?"

Since women are so often victims of violence, Pat knew it was essential for each and every ER to have a policy of asking all victims questions about their injuries and to know different types of injuries and recognize the kind that most likely result from violence. Often, as with Judy, there would be a history of minor complaints, of crying out for help. When that cry for help was not recognized, other symptoms were sure to follow.

"My minister told me that we should never have married in the first place," a tearful Judy said. "He said

I should just leave. He doesn't realize what it's like to be alone in the world with two kids to support.

"Another therapist we went to for counseling said that maybe I needed to stay home more and make sure I was a proper wife. But I *was* a proper wife. He told me not to argue with my husband." She wiped the tears away. "But I was never the one to start the arguments. He would, over the slightest things, like a dish that didn't sparkle when I set his place for dinner." She described how, when she had, one time, inadvertently put a knife out with a water spot, he had been so incensed that he had kicked over the table, food and all. He constantly brought up that she was a failure because of her first divorce; that, even though she only weighed 120 pounds at 5'6", she was too fat, that the baby cried too much, and that she was an unfit mother.

No matter what she did, nothing was good enough for her husband. This is because abusers keep changing the rules to suit their own needs. If they want to pick a fight, they will find something to be upset about, even if previously the same situation had not upset them.

She wasn't even sure she wanted to stay married anymore, but with two children she didn't think she had a choice at the moment.

Judy had tried to leave once, before she had become pregnant. She had been homeless and on the street with her daughter from her first marriage, forced to beg for food from their church. He put every conceivable pressure on her to bring her back, and in the end she had returned to him.

Once Judy allowed her husband to come for a hospital visit, he started trying to take control. He demanded the right to talk to her doctor and staff.

Judy was clearly cowed when she saw him. He acted as if it was his due. Kissing her and hugging her, he came with gifts enough to make almost any woman swoon. Judy was no exception. She glanced at the nurse, as if to say, "See, he really does love me."

Tension continued through the visit. Judy responded a bit more to him, but she was still stiff in the presence of her husband. They spoke in Armenian. Pat was sure it was so that she would not know what they were saying and interfere.

When he had left, Judy told her, "He wants me to come back. He says things will be different now. That he didn't know just how I was feeling."

"And do you believe him? Do you want to return?"

"I don't know. I don't know." Judy wrung her hands with indecision. "I want to have a good home for Kara, the baby, and myself. I don't know what to do. What do you think?" she asked tearfully.

"I think no human has a right to treat another human the way you tell me your husband has treated you. No one should be subjected to name calling and to violence at the whim of another person."

"I know, but I love him . . . I think."

"I can't tell you what to do, Judy. Only you can

make that decision. But someone who loves you should not be treating you like that."

As Pat continued to reinforce with Judy what a good relationship was, Judy became stronger.

As soon as Judy was able to handle it, Pat lined her up with a battered women's group that had Armenian workers, so she would not feel so isolated. With the help of Pat and the shelter, Judy filed for a restraining order and a divorce and was set up on welfare with the Violence Against Women program, which provided for money and food stamps and housing subsidy in some states for an unlimited time to women who are victims of domestic abuse.

The only way to break such a cycle as this is to be proactive. Pat hoped that she had gotten to the family in time to prevent the daughters from seeking abusive love relationships in the future.

Since women are so often the victims of violence, it is essential that women who present themselves to emergency departments for even minor trauma be thoroughly evaluated. ED staff must be aware of the types of injuries most likely resulting from violence, and the victim must be asked about the cause of the trauma to determine if it is the result of violence and whether further evaluation is required.

Until recently, it was thought that the marriage gave the husband total license to use the woman and her body any time and in any way he desired it. Declaring that your husband raped you was not an accepted complaint. Now, however, several states have made it a crime to force anyone, even your wife, to have sexual relations against her will.

Domestic violence victims who report rape by their intimate partners experience a significant drop in self-esteem as opposed to those who do not report it. Partners who rape their significant others are more violent and dish out more emotional abuse. They are also more likely to kill their partners. So, if a woman has reported rape by her partner, the likelihood of his attempting to kill her increases. Any threat against her needs to be taken seriously by the law, because too often it is not.

Women have a hard time believing the person they fell in love with will kill them. Unfortunately, it happens all the time.

If the victim is alone, the SANE will talk with her about whom she would like to call and where she will go from the hospital. Every effort will be made to find a place for her to go where she will feel safe and will not be alone. When necessary, arrangements may be made for shelter placement.

If she is intoxicated or does not want to leave until morning, arrangements may be made for her to sleep in a specified area of the hospital when this type of space is available.

A battered woman's advocate is often on the SART team, since many women are raped by their partners. Because of this, the sexual assault teams need to be aware of the domestic abuse policy at their hospital and need to be aware not only of stranger rapes but marital rapes as well.

Domestic violence is the perpetuation of violent acts by one individual on another, whether that act is psychological or physical. Recently, definitions of domestic violence and/or child abuse started including children witnessing violent incidents in the home, since those children are exposed to the psychological effects of seeing that happen. Children witnessing such an act may ultimately act out against the abuser and/or become abusers themselves.

The children suffer further psychological damage when the parents talk negatively about each other. The control issues continue. If we look at police reports, many tell of the children being used to threaten the other parent. The children become pawns in the relationship. Frequently the courts do not enforce restraining orders or court orders as they should. A restraining order is generally in place when the tension and/or violence has escalated and/or one of the parties makes actual or perceived threats against the other.

Restraining orders are legal orders telling the persons involved in these incidents to stay away from each other. That legal order may or may not be enforceable. Until recently, these orders were difficult to enforce without returning to the court that issued them. In order to provide adequate protection, a restraining order or order of protection must be enforceable at the street level. Enforcement at the street level can take immediate action to remove the offending party, thereby reducing the injuries seen in domestic incidents.

Another major issue in domestic violence is the lack of ability to get out of the situation.

Until recently, local law enforcement officers were unable to enforce restraining orders. There have been numerous homicides in which there was a restraining order in place and local law enforcement officials could not enforce it.

The role of the forensic nurse in answering a domestic violence call is to assess and judge, provide information, and make arrangements for follow-up for transportation to shelters, arrange for care of children if both parents are arrested. This needs to be done as quickly as possible. Since the laws may or may not be clearly defined, it is the responsibility of the law enforcement officer to determine any legal charges and arrests to be made. The dynamics of domestic violence must be recognized. There may be mandatory arrest policies in the jurisdiction that the nurse needs to be aware of. The response needs to be a team effort. Injury assessment by the nurse and notification of EMS as needed or at the request of the victim should be a priority.

On calls, there needs to be a good understanding of each person's role and what to do if the call goes bad. The officer can't be expected to spend time worrying about the nurse if the assailant returns—each person needs to know what to do and when to do it. Each team member needs to be able to trust one another and work as one. Self-defense training can help build teamwork and confidence as well.

If nurses will be answering service calls in the field with the officers, there needs to be very clear role delineation. The officer is in charge at the scene. The officer should be the one to determine whether or not the scene is safe enough to proceed. If it appears that the conditions are not safe to do an assessment and documentation, either the victim needs to be transported to a place of safety or arrangements need to be made to do the documentation at another location or at a later time. If contact is made out in the field (as in response to police calls), the time should be kept as brief as possible. Documentation should include narrative, body maps, and photos. Assessment will be brief and must be objective. If the setting is a clinic, more time will be available. These same general principles apply in the clinical setting. Often assailants come to visit victims and the staff needs to know what to do if this should occur. Information on safety, resources, and shelters needs to be given to the victim. Ideally, a victim advocate will also be on-site to discuss issues of obtaining a restraining order or order of protection, seeking shelter, legal options, resources, and child issues. The nurse needs to define her role as objective forensic documentation of injuries. The nurse may also offer the victim information about safety, safety planning, and legal assistance, but needs to remain objective. One of the biggest areas missing in this field is the documentation of injuries to the alleged assailant. Judges see a need for this, so that when the case does go to court, both sides have documentation. This would be a role for the nurse as well. If the role is defined as objective forensic documentation of injuries, this would benefit all involved. There is a need for follow-up photos. Bruising may not be visible in its full array of color at the time of injury. Follow-up photos and documentation, as well as use of alternate light source photography (that potentially show the underlying areas of bruising or injury) are very beneficial. Careful assessment for head injury as well as strangulation is imperative. Again, documentation by photos, narrative, and body maps must be done in a concise, clear, and objective manner. Court training should be done by the local prosecutor's office and should include applicable laws, courtroom observation, mock trial, and court etiquette.

Legislation is needed at all levels, from prevention to incarceration, to deal with domestic violence. What constitutes domestic violence in a particular jurisdiction needs to be clearly defined by law.

Nurses are in an excellent position to promote legislation. They are taught to gather information (including statistical) and present findings and conclusions. We need to talk to representatives at a personal level and tell them how we see the problem in our community. They need to be informed, so that they are better able to represent the needs of the community and propose solutions to these problems.

A good starting point for a nurse wishing to establish a domestic violence team is to gather statistics and form a multiagency task force that includes community members. Information available or the lack of available information is a good indicator of the needs in the community and resources in place. The statistical information can provide a picture of what is currently going on in the community in the jurisdiction. Public awareness is essential. Involvement of the media with accurate information and public resources will provide awareness of the problem and support for the response team. Response to domestic violence involves the entire community. Nurses are in a unique position to collect and interpret statistical information, work with agencies and interdisciplinary teams, document forensic evidence, create response teams, and promote change.

The Criminally Insane

"Are you sure you want to work with forensic psychiatry?" The interviewer was astonished. It was clear he didn't get too many nurses asking to be transferred to the mental health unit housing the offenders who had pleaded insanity.

"Sure," Eva said.

"John Hinkley is there. You know, the guy who tried to kill President Reagan."

"Oh, yeah, I know that," the nurse said.

"You know you always have to be on your guard for unpredictable behavior. They'll try to manipulate the hell out of you."

"What else is new? Psychiatric patients are often like that."

"Some of these guys appeared pretty normal until they . . ." The interviewer made a cutthroat sign.

"Yes," Eva persisted. "I want to work there." She

smiled. "Don't worry. I have relatives in law enforcement, and my ex-boyfriend's a homicide cop."

He shook his head. "We have a hard time getting nurses to come on this unit. You really are sure?"

"I really am sure."

Psychiatric nursing in criminal institutions is one of the original forms of forensic nursing. Since the mid-1800s, nurses have taken care of convicts or offenders who have pleaded insanity, or whose competence to stand trial is in question. As a profession, it started in the United Kingdom with the advent of Broadmoor Special Hospital for the Criminally Insane, and started with perpetrators rather than victims. Even within this role, there are diverse subspecialties, some with their own unique therapies.

The idea of forensic nurses dealing with victims is a recent phenomenon.

In England, Europe, and Canada, when you talk about forensic nurses, most of them are forensic psychiatric or correctional nurses. Outside the United States, schools that teach forensic nursing concentrate mainly on psychiatry and/or correctional nursing (caring for the convicts in the jail system).

Nurses working in prisons, similar to those working in forensic psychiatry, must be able to put their moral judgments behind them. They have to look past the offense and the offender to give good medical care to their patients.

"I had worked in the emergency room for eight

years and I never thought of it as being forensic," says Arlene.

"By this time in my career, I needed a change. I looked for something different and happened on a relief job at the jail. I really liked it. I thought it was nursing's best-kept secret. I found the work challenging and multidimensional, like the ER had been, but with more autonomy. The population [of prisoners] fascinated me, especially their behavior, and the stresses they were under and understanding how they came to be in this situation. I worked at the remand center for three more years and then transferred to the forensic psychiatry department at the nearby general hospital and remained there many years."

Forensic psychiatry is like asking which came first—the chicken or the egg. Did the offender become crazy after he committed the crime? Or was he already crazy and was the crime a result of his paranoia? Did the drugs he took induce the psychosis, or did he have it already and they only pushed him over the edge?

To put it more simply, if a person killed his landlord, did he kill him because voices or a paranoia told him to do it, or did the horrific events of his crime drive him crazy? If he had been on medications before, did he stop taking them? Did he imagine some wrong that became magnified until the only thing he felt he could do was murder?

"Making assessments and evaluations of the patient-offender is challenging, at best. If they are on the forensic psychiatric unit, it is because they have a legal charge against them and the court wants to see if they are fit to stand trial. We see every type of psychiatric dysfunction on our unit, it's just that there is a legal aspect to their care, as well," Arlene says.

"We're required to provide a letter to the court so that they can understand what is happening to that person at this time in their life. This gives them more information when deciding about sentencing. Although we give recommendations, it's not our job to judge right from wrong. Sometimes, it's just a matter of getting them regulated on their medications, which they might have stopped."

Recognized as an expert witness, Arlene has appeared before the court a few different times as a consultant in independent cases. Working full-time in clinical practice, Arlene felt the need to write about what forensic nurses do. "I knew I needed more education before I could achieve any kind of international credibility in that area." She continues to pursue a doctorate in forensic nursing.

One of the Canadian board members of IAFN, Arlene is responsible for encouraging Mount Royal College to develop an on-site and Internet course for forensic nurses. Arlene now uses many years of practice to draw from when developing, writing, and teaching forensic nursing courses. Some of the courses are overviews and others concentrate on a subgenre of forensic nursing. She has held a classroom forensic nursing course at the University of Calgary every spring since 1995, two online courses at Mount Royal

College since 1997, and is currently developing courses for Athabasca University.

John, a former police officer turned nurse, does forensic psychiatry, working with the perpetrators in the state hospital for the criminally insane. It's a city within a city. "I knew I could make a difference there," he says. "Most of the nurses working there didn't know anything about law enforcement. I had a different viewpoint. I knew about the criminal mind a bit differently. I was able to teach them from my combined experience.

"As nurses, we want to cure and help everyone, but there are no medications to fix antisocial personalities."

John is also one of those called to court to testify if he believes the person is still a danger to self or society, often called a "5150." "You can fool a doctor for a few hours, but you can't fool the nurses who talk to and observe the criminally insane for fifteen hours a day, seven days a week. It's really hard to keep that kind of act up. They don't get away. When they are released from us, that means that they are well enough to stand trial and often return to prison."

Working with verbal judo or tactical communication, John knows how to get difficult people to do what he wants. He was taught this as a police officer and passes his expertise on to his fellow nurses.

"We had a 254-pound guy, Sunny, who, standing at six-foot-four, was barricaded in his room armed with a metal mop wringer and a plan to take out the first person coming in through the door. I was called.

" 'I can see you're upset, Sunny,' I said. 'But what you're planning isn't going to happen.' I referred to his plan to kill someone because he was upset at not getting the meal he wanted. 'I'm going to order the towels and water now.' I motioned to the security guard who stood behind me now.

" 'For what?' Sunny asked, suspiciously.

" 'Well, if I can't talk to you, then the police will come. They'll spray you and it will burn.'

"After that, Sunny, who had been known on the ward for his unpredictable behavior, for breaking down seclusion doors and tearing apart restraints, was like a puppy.

"I let him know that I would respect him if he would respect me. There were only two people on the ward that day.

"He let him come in. He calmed down without an incident. Later that day, I was writing in the charts at the desk. He came to the door of the office.

" 'Can I talk to you, John?'

" 'Sure, Sunny. Just let me finish this chart. Give me five minutes.'

" 'Fuck five minutes. I want to talk to you now.'

" 'Not if you talk to me like that. I know you're upset, because otherwise you would never talk like that.' (He talked like that all the time.)

"It was like letting steam out of a balloon. I couldn't believe the change that came over Sunny. 'Yeah, sure. Okay. Five minutes.' He was now willing and compliant. 'You writing a good note about me?'

" 'Yes, I am writing about what happened.' I closed the chart. 'Okay, I'm ready. Let's go talk.' I led him out to the day room.

"This technique has really cut down on the number of problems we've seen. The idea is putting yourself in their shoes and trying to see things from their viewpoint. We want to get through the moment without hurting anyone. You can't personalize what is going on. We are staff. I just want to leave at the end of the day and feel safe, and know that the other staff are safer for what I've done."

When he was a kid, ballistics was one of John's hobbies, but he doesn't profess to be an expert in that. "I get called to testify all the time on behavior and individuals, but I don't consider myself an expert witness. I just try to learn as much as I can so that I can tell others what is going on, as I see it."

Sometimes John finds the best thing to do is become a victim advocate. He feels one of the best ways for nurses and police to understand each other is to "walk a thousand miles in their moccasins." He suggests ride-alongs, learning each other's terminology, having the police spend a few shifts in the ER. "The more we know about each other's job and responsibilities, the more we can respect and appreciate each other. We are all on the same team, it's just a matter of playing the same game.

"On almost every ride-along I have gone on, I have picked up on something the cops did not. They wouldn't even have known what to look for. That's the advantage of the forensic nurse who is cross-trained. I know the rules about touching, I know that the officer is doing the actual investigation, but I can look at an injury and say that it doesn't make sense, it doesn't jibe with the story. The borders of the abrasion, the direction that the abrasion is traveling, or the skin tags all tell me a story that is different from what the victim is saying. In several instances, the officers went back in after I examined the situation, and the guy admitted that my version of his story was correct.

"Other times, the officers thought the person was high on something. I would look in the medicine cabinet and see a prescription drug that would give the same effect."

There are usually two different sectors of NGBRI (Not Guilty by Reason of Insanity) units. One for pretrial, to determine if the offender is competent to stand trial, and the other for those already sentenced but who, in the eyes of the court, lack the mental capacity to understand fully that what they did is wrong.

The definition of sanity differs greatly, depending on whether you are talking to a doctor or a lawyer, and it's a fine line that the courts have to walk in determining the best location for an inmate.

The fact that our landlord killer knew it was wrong makes him sane in some eyes; the fact that he heard voices telling him to kill makes him insane in others.

As one might expect, the patients in the NGBRI units are more resistant to treatment than the usual psych inpatient. Once they are "sane," they return to the mainstream of jail.

Many of them stay in denial for as long as the system will allow them to stay in psych, but the discharge goals are the same: to get them functional in daily life.

"You are not making them well to go home," Pat, another forensic psychiatric nurse, says. "You are teaching them to modify their behavior and give them certain skills to survive the years they have left to serve in prison. Face it, the child molester can't be cured."

The laws of states vary and allow the offenders between sixty days and their full term, depending on the state and county. Most will stay for evaluation and treatment until they have proven themselves no longer dangerous to themselves or others. For some of the offenders, that's their lifetime, unless they can manipulate the system to be released. Often they will just go on to other hospitals.

"In the early seventies and eighties, there were a lot of misdiagnoses due to alcohol and drugs. There were a lot of critically mentally ill in the prison system and vice versa. Quite a few of the people I treated at the mental health clinic belonged in jail. They knew right from wrong and just did not want to take responsibility."

Barbara is a forensic nurse who works independently of the jail system, informally assisting the legal system in making decisions about competency. She works both in the unsentenced program (those who have been arraigned) and with those who have already been found at fault. With a master's in psychiatric nursing, she has two nurses working under her and she assigns cases based on her staff at hand. She finds that a team approach works best.

A lot of mental illness can be successfully treated from within the jail. Most jails have psychiatrists associated with them who come and see the offenders on a weekly basis and check on their medications. To put someone in the forensic psychiatric unit costs over $700 per day.

The interviews she does are usually conducted because the judge has had a question after how the offender behaved in court, though most murder and large drug cases are reviewed.

Louis was referred to Barbara's office by a judge who wanted certain questions answered. Among them: Was Louis fit and ready to stand trial? Did he understand what he had done? Did he know that it was wrong?

"After interviewing Louis, my first step was to gather all his medical and hospital records," Barbara says. "I had to decide what had come first, the mental illness or the substance abuse problem.

" 'Louis, do you know why you're here?'

"He nodded and grinned, showing his nicotine-stained teeth. 'I was a bad boy.'

" 'What did you do that was bad?'

"He shrugged and looked up toward the corner of the room. I looked there, too, wondering what he was seeing. Obviously, he was responding to some internal stimuli. I certainly hoped his voices weren't saying anything about me. His history, until the violent episode when he had lashed out at his mother, was one of passivity. But it was hard to know what might push someone over the edge.

"Louis had all the signs of mental illness. He hallucinated, exhibited behavior that was out of order, and had been in and out of mental and rehab programs. Having worked over eight years in the jail system, I can pretty much tell when they're telling me the truth and when they are lying. If I have any doubts, I will ask the same question over and over again, until something clicks or until they trip up and say something inconsistent with their prior story. I continued with my mental status exam.

" 'Louis, what did you do that was bad?' I asked again.

"He gave a little laugh, almost as if he was talking to himself. I could just imagine him, sitting on the pee-stained sofa in his mother's house, long greasy hair dragging in his face, laughing to some other-worldly joke.

" 'Louis, do you know where we are?'

" 'Hospital,' he mumbled.

" 'Who's the president, Louis?'

" 'Of the world?' He blinked as he asked me. I turned around again because he seemed to be staring at something just above my shoulder, but there was nothing there.

" 'No, Louis, of the United States.'

" 'Oh, yeah. That one. Uh . . . Clinton.' He made a lewd gesture with his hips and grinned.

"I didn't know if that meant he was up on the news or not. 'Right. Clinton. Do you know what day it is?'

" 'Tu . . . Tuesday.'

"He was close. It was Wednesday. Two out of three wasn't bad, but either he didn't want to or couldn't yet talk about his mother's death.

"After several more questions, I dismissed Louis for the day and sat down to check out his records.

"In the past, people did not really investigate the health history of the individuals being sentenced. I found a reference to Louis's drinking nearly fifteen years earlier, as well as a mention of a violent outburst against another patient who had taken one of Louis's cigarettes. He had been on and off numerous antipsychotic medications for most of his life. The day treatment program he had attended charted that they were seeing some erratic behavior. A good indication that Louis had, perhaps, stopped taking his medication on a regular basis as he should have been.

"Louis was due back at court in a week's time, but it seemed pretty clear-cut to me that he needed hospitalization, and that was what I would recommend. I doubted Louis would change much even with treatment. The best we could hope for would be to keep him from hurting himself or others. Too often the public expects miracles from the psychiatric system, which it just can't deliver.

"Kevin, on the other hand, whom I had interviewed

that morning, and who claimed to be hearing voices, had his answers too pat to be believable. However, he did have a history of drug abuse, which could be a part of his problem. I had to research his records and see what the history said on him before I made my decision. I had to remember that most of the patients in forensic psychiatry have personality disorders, often exhibit antisocial behaviors, some are just outright psychotic. More than 70 percent of them are prone to violence and acting out, so just being violent, in and of itself, does not count as being crazy.

"Even if a person is psychotic when they commit a crime, you can't overlook that a crime has been committed and there is still a victim.

"Most of the offenders are very good at saying what they think you want to hear. In forensic psychiatry, you have to learn not to take what they say at face value.

"I didn't have the last say on any of the cases; after I made my report, the psychiatrist would interview them, as well, and do formal hearings, but my recommendation saved him time. As a nurse, I also have to understand the criminal justice system in our state, since the legal definition of competency is different from the medical one. Therefore, it's the judge who makes the final decision. After that, the Bureau of Forensics decides where they go.

"In order to write a good report, you have to be able to talk to the judge in both lay and legal terms. The first part the nurses can do, the second is harder. But it's like the mountain and Mohammed. We have to go to them and learn their language, because very few of them learn ours.

"Francis was an eighty-six-year-old man who had done a mercy killing on his wife, Ilene. She suffered from cancer. He, himself, suffered from high blood pressure and heart problems. I got a call from security.

" 'Barb, you got to get this guy out of here. We can't handle him. He's got too many medical problems. He's getting on our nerves. Someone's gonna kill him.'

" 'Why? What's wrong?'

" 'He's just not taking care of himself. He's not washing, he's not dressing, and he's not . . .'

" 'In other words, he's not doing his ADLs, activities of daily living.'

" 'Yeah, that, too.'

"Not taking care of oneself is one of the signs of depression, but depression is something that goes along with being in prison. Not many people are happy about spending time inside. If he were suicidal, I could have done something, but he wasn't.

" 'I know, his attorney called me. He wants him out of there just because of his age. He thinks someone will harm Francis. But my problem is that he is formally competent. The man has no psychiatric history and no need for mental health treatment. Why should I sentence him to dealing with these patients?'

"Francis, however, was determined to deteriorate. He refused to do anything. He never left his cell even for meals.

"During the formal company hearing, Francis was obviously having trouble breathing. His congestive heart failure was worsening. 'Take him to the hospital,' our doctor ordered. Francis's competency hearing would be postponed until he had stabilized.

"Two weeks later, the judge asked me to pay Francis a visit in the hospital and do an informal competency hearing to see how the old man was doing. 'Can you believe it,' the judge told me, 'the DA still wants to press charges?'

"I could see that Francis was in a lot of pain both from his arthritis and his congestive heart failure.

" 'I'm going to plead not guilty,' he wheezed.

"I let him know that when we went back to court, if he could not answer the judge's questions, he would be judged incompetent.

"So we went back to court as soon as the medical doctor had cleared Francis. He didn't say a word. He refused to answer any questions." He died in custody a few months later.

"Cecil was a twenty-four-year-old man who totally refused to cooperate with his attorney in court, and so a formal competency hearing was ordered," Barbara tells another story.

" 'He needs a drug rehab,' I told the judge.

"We began looking for a treatment place for him and went back to court.

"Almost immediately the attorney objected to my report.

"I pointed to the bottom line where it said that I was the mental health expert the court had chosen. Then I explained to him that the reason Cecil was not cooperating with the attorney or with drug rehab placement was because he was using drugs in jail.

" 'You know that for a fact?' the judge asked me.

"I nodded. I produced the results of the tests we had taken on him and pointed out the behavior changes that the guards and other inmates had reported over the past few weeks. 'Besides,' I told the judge, 'my sources at the jail give me reports, which back up what we have here.' "

Barbara, who serves as an expert witness for several courts and also sits on review boards, is currently working on a glossary of psychiatric terms to give to the juries so that they can understand what bipolar (manic-depressive) is and what schizophrenia is. "If the jury understands what we are doing, then they can understand how we came to our opinions. It gives us more credibility."

Some hospitals have separate wings for the forensic patients, others are totally independent.

"There are times when the crimes committed are just so horrible you wonder how anyone sane could do them, but they do," Pat says. "All the same, we don't usually get Hannibal Lectors. That type of serial killer seldom ends up in the psychiatric units. People can be evil, and they do evil things with bad intent merely because they want to, and not because they are crazy."

Forty-year-old Richard looked like a CPA—slender, studious, sparse dark hair over his balding crown, and glasses. He acted like one, too, seldom raising his voice above the sound of a whisper, and just so polite.

This same man bludgeoned his twin five-year-old daughters to death with a sledgehammer. His first story was that he had lost them in a store. Then he claimed to have had a blackout, sort of a fugue state, and that he really meant to kill himself with the sledgehammer. But he made a choice to go down into that basement.

The psychiatrist believed him. Pat did not. Because they disagreed, he was discharged back to jail after eighty-four days in the psychiatric ward and went to face the charges. "After all," Pat told the doctor, "he's no longer a threat to himself." His suicidal thoughts had obviously passed. And he obviously understood the case against him. They could have recommended that he stay at the hospital, but it was pretty obvious that he was just using them because he thought the psychiatric ward was a better place than jail.

Almost everyone in jail and in the forensic psychiatric ward would have you believe they are innocent. You ask them what their charges are, and they will tell you, "Well, the cops said I did this and this, but I didn't." You have to look past that and see what the facts are. No one goes out to rob a bank and plans on getting caught. And if they do, they assume they're going to beat the rap.

Probably the biggest population at Pat's place is sexual offenders. Sam was a truck driver and a chameleon. Like Richard, he initially came off as being soft-spoken and quiet. "He kept to himself. We had no problems with him. I was beginning to think that a mistake had been made by sending him to our unit," Pat says. "I have to admit that even I was taken in by him. When dealing with these people, you have to be realistic and just observe. Be quiet, be nonjudgmental, and observe the facts as the facts. Sam ended up sending chills through me, and, considering what I have seen and heard, few people do that."

Sam's case was particularly gruesome. He kidnapped a young boy, molested him, and threw him out of his truck at high speed into the freezing water. Thinking him dead, he sped away. The kid survived, barely.

"As soon as we went back to court and Sam knew that he was being extradited to Pennsylvania, the pretense was over," Pat says. "We saw a different side of him then. No sooner did we return to the unit than he struck up an acquaintance with one of our other patients. Bart was nineteen but he looked a lot younger, and Sam was a pedophile.

" "We watched, unable to do much but try and keep the two separated, as with giddy, juvenile, lovesick behavior he bonded the young man to him. The change was almost overnight. When the barber came, Sam shaved off his eyebrows and head so that he would look younger. There was nothing psychotic about him, it was pure evil intent.

"Sam ended up escaping from the unit transporting

him and went out west to murder a couple of people in California.

"Some people just can't be rehabilitated. I think after ten years working in forensic psychiatry, I am more for the death penalty than I was before. It's not just retribution. You have to protect the majority, and sometimes death is the only way. Even if the offender is deemed crazy, there is always a crime and always a victim."

It's not only men who are in the forensic psychiatry wards. Women get sent there, too, though most of them have been sexually and physically abused and most of them have kids.

Occasionally, the forensic nurses have someone who is so sick and disorganized that they have no idea why they did something, like the eighteen-year-old girl who had come back to her family, delivered a baby, and threw it in the trash. The baby was still alive, but died shortly after. To the mother's mind, the baby had been dead already.

To some people, a nurse is a nurse is a nurse, but that is not always the case. Unique skills are needed for handling each area of nursing, as they are for handling each area of forensic nursing.

Even working as a psychiatric nurse in a regular ward, Joan found she was encountering many clients who had legal as well as medical issues.

In 1995, as an aftermath of the Lucasville, Ohio,

riot, the inmates sued Governor Voinovich. The outcome of the lawsuit was that the Ohio Department of Rehabilitation and Corrections would develop its own mental health services in Ohio prisons.

As the Department of Mental Health's primary oversight person, Joan now takes a very active role in forensic psychiatric nursing, trying to get the forensic nurse accepted as a specialist with unique education and special skills. Just because someone is skilled in psychiatry, Joan found out, it doesn't mean that they can handle forensic psychiatry.

"There are extra skills that you don't think about when you are working in forensic psychiatry or in corrections. Security is a big issue, and so is boundary setting. You can't go and hug a patient here, like you might in a regular, open ward. You have to learn to give your support through eye contact and voice tone. You have to give care without appearing to be judgmental or cold, and with some of these offenders, that's a real trick."

As many nurses, Jeanette went into nursing to help people. Having done a psychiatry practicum at the prison, she found she liked the diversity. "I had been thinking of becoming a social worker to help the troubled youth, but I realized I could accomplish something in the jails, too. I proved to the authorities that if we increased the self-esteem of the prisoners, it would make their job easier, they would cause fewer problems, and, hopefully, they would not reoffend. Although they are in prison against their will, you still have to deliver medical care to them."

The corrections nurse has much more independence than the hospital nurse, probably because there are fewer of them. It also means they have to use their own resources.

"The offenders quickly learn not to bite the hand that feeds them, and the older ones often keep the younger ones in line. That's not to say they won't try to play one staff member against another, or try to manipulate the hell out of you, but they do try to protect you.

"Once," Jeanette relates, "when I was a young staff member, the inmates told me and my coworker to stay on the other unit. They knew unrest was at hand and they were protecting us. They wouldn't tell us directly, but they alluded to it, and we took the hint."

Despite the impression that some might have, of them just passing pills, the corrections nurses have to be alert to forensic implications of events as well.

During a period of unrest, the nurses were especially busy with checking on injured inmates. When Kevin, a convicted child molester, came into the medical unit after complaining that one of the guards had attacked him and stabbed him, Jeanette examined the wound and took photos for the file.

No matter who had stabbed him, it could easily develop into a legal case.

She was surprised to note that, for a stab wound, both edges seemed too clean. Jeanette pointed out to the warden that, in fact, the weapon used on Kevin was probably homemade by one of the inmates, since those making knives illicitly on the unit usually sharpened both sides as best they could.

The guard who had been accused of the incident was grateful not to lose his job.

The nurses working in corrections not only do psychiatric assessments but have to deal with medical emergencies as well.

Sherry was called to the women's jail because one of the new female officers had noticed that an inmate's underwear and jeans were wet when she was being changed into her jail jumpsuit. The inmate, Karen, was supposedly seven months pregnant.

Sherry listened to the fetal heart tones. They seemed regular but she suspected premature rupture of the membranes.

"Have you done anything that might affect your pregnancy?"

"Nope."

"No drugs, no alcohol . . ."

Karen shook her head. "Nothing, nurse."

Karen appeared to be speaking coherently but quietly.

Not wanting to make a mistake in case it was a rupture of the membranes, Sherry called for the van to take her to the ER.

Minutes went by.

Karen began to mumble. Her speech was slurring,

and she was, in general, decompensating and appeared to be under the influence.

"You sure she didn't take drugs?" the female officer asked.

"What's her charges?" Sherry asked.

"Drugs," the officer said, looking at the computer screen. "But she turned herself in when she found out about the warrant."

Sherry looked at the patient's arms. There were no needle tracks, but Karen was becoming worse. Worried that the van had not yet arrived, Sherry called the ambulance just as Karen went into premature labor. It turned out that Karen, knowing she was going in, had loaded up on narcotics.

The patient was airlifted to the medical center, since the baby was still very small. With the help of the officer in charge of the women's jail, Sherry and the other people involved filed child endangerment charges. The baby, as soon as it was born, would be taken into a protected environment.

Thanks to the officer's observation and the nurse's work, the child's life was saved.

Often after going to court and being publicly accused of his alleged crimes, the offender comes back to the jail very depressed.

Sherry was called into the holding room because Eugene, a man who had been convicted of 350 counts of child molestation and child pornography, was suicidal.

Agitated and depressed, he began talking to Sherry. He was anxious that he would be convicted for the full forty years. He was over forty now. He feared he would never make it out alive. Overwhelmed with fears about his future, his worldly goods that still remained in his apartment, and how he would handle his idle time once he was permanently placed, not to mention what would greet him in prison, he just could not cope.

"When arrested, he had been working as a character actor for children's birthday parties," Sherry says. "A well-built, good-looking man, with a mustache and goatee, he probably could have passed for a thinner Colonel Sanders. I remember hearing the officers talking about how physically ill they had become during the investigation, seeing in his apartment the home videos of Eugene having sex with the children.

"I knew that within a few days the paper would be full of the court proceedings and of the victims relating how Eugene had ruined their lives.

"As he talked to me, he downplayed his activities, blaming anything he could think of, including the Internet. 'You know, I was once a nurse, myself. I have a bachelor's degree,' he said, trying to put us on an equal level. 'How am I supposed to handle all this?' "

Like many forensic nurses, Sherry had a skill of compartmentalizing—that is, putting her personal feelings to one side while she became an active listener and problem solver for the perpetrator. She had used the skill when doing sexual assault exams, when going to crime scenes, and when assisting with autopsies.

The ability was even more crucial in corrections, because the nurse is called upon so often to help those that society despises.

"As I sat down with Eugene, I heard a man overwhelmed with grief, sadness, despair, and maybe a touch of remorse and guilt. We started with listing his material possessions, since it's easier for people to start with concrete things. Then we progressed to who would take care of his things on the outside, and what needed to be done.

"I had him put on suicide watch, and, for a week, I could see him writing his lists and lightening up, feeling that his chores were being taken care of."

In Canada's province of British Columbia, they have now instituted a position called Forensic Liaison Office. Julia is one of these. A nurse with the local mental health services, she is considered a friend of the crown (or court). However, she speaks both for the client and for the crown.

It's Julia's job to establish and identify risk in the adult population. Another nurse with the Ministry of Children handles the juveniles. Using Dr. Hart's Weber and Weber HCR20 exam, she sorts out those with predisposition for problems and connects them with the various services and does case management. Anyone suffering from a mental disorder and having a criminal charge is sent to Julia.

"Each individual is a different situation and has different needs, which must be met." She has, however, found a lot more substance abuse and associated problems in the forensic population.

"One of the main differences between forensic psychiatry and the regular psychiatry is the profiles you see. We get more pedophiles and sex offenders than the general population of psychiatric clients. And I have to stomach a lot of criminal behavior, concentrating on the person and not what he has done.

"We get manipulated more, too. As a nurse, I have to believe everything they say, and nothing at all. I check out almost all that the offenders tell me.

"When Art called me up, crying about how much he loved his wife, how much he wanted her back, I reminded him of how he treated her and of his restraining order. Then he threatened suicide. 'I never did anything wrong to her. She forced me to leave. God, you have to believe me. I love her so much. I never harmed her. I love her too much, I would have never touched her. It was all a misunderstanding. I just want to die without her. If I can't have her back, I will kill myself. I know I will.'

"After a severe beating, which left her hospitalized, he was taken to prison, where he tried to hang himself.

"Rescued in what appeared to be the nick of time, he again professed his love for his ex-wife and his determination to be with her again and to 'just work things out like we ought to have done.'

"He was taken to the forensic psychiatric ward for an evaluation.

"The psychiatrist, taken in, was about to put him in touch with his ex-wife, when I handed him the police report detailing her cuts, bruises, and broken bones. It detailed how she lost her baby after he throttled her, claiming that she had been fooling around with other men (which she denied ever doing).

"Dr. See wasn't the only one who believed Art. Almost everyone on the ward did, after his pseudo–suicide attempt. Neither the doctor nor the ward staff had read the police reports in the file. The other staff had bought into his distraction and his denial, forgetting who he really was and why he was in the forensic psychiatric ward.

"When his ruse failed, he admitted that he really did not intend to kill himself, but he would like to kill his ex-wife.

"As a forensic nurse, I have to be suspicious of everyone and everything. I have to know his personality and understand the profile—in this case, of the abuser," Julia says.

While society has long used the nurse in the correction facilities and in hospitals, it is only within the last two decades that the forensic psychiatric nurse has been recognized for the vital role that she plays in the care and rehabilitation of prisoners and the mentally ill who have committed crimes. Her opinions and views, which were once dismissed, are now given weight in the court and respected as those given by somebody constantly caring for and observing the patients.

The forensic nurse started from this humble beginning in the United Kingdom, and then developed further by nurses here in the United States who were not only advocates of the patients but advocates of justice as well; nurses who thought there could be a better way to help patients tell their stories and nurses who felt they had to be the voices for those who could not talk and those who could no longer tell their stories; nurses who saw that they could assist police with their observations; nurses who were not intimidated by the prosecuting "sharks." These nurses have all learned the silent language of evidence that tells the tale, even when the victims or perpetrators cannot.

Despite shows like *CSI,* our crime labs are very understaffed. We, the forensic nurses, ask your help to support the Paul Coverdell National Forensic Sciences Improvement Act to give more and updated equipment to labs and to also support programs and hospitals that use forensic nurses.

Acknowledgments

Last but not least in this book is the story of Virginia Lynch, the woman who has, almost single-handedly, brought forensic nursing in all its manifestations to America's health service. Lecturing with fire and brimstone, this Southern belle has spread her message not only through the United States, but across the globe. It's been her vision and her energy that has stimulated others to go ahead with their goals. She has motivated them to return home to their own communities determined to make a difference in the way we work with police and in the way evidence is collected.

Virginia's own training was trial and error. Her transformation went from ignorant student, knowing nothing about the surroundings of death, to one who specialized in it. There were no nurses helping her through the grief process when a family member died.

Working in the ER she would see evidence and not

know the meaning of it. When she failed to collect it properly, the police and district attorneys would be upset. She asked what needed to be done but they didn't know how to answer her.

So Virginia headed straight to the source. At the crime lab she asked them to instruct her on how to collect the evidence that was useable in their cases.

She started out first in forensic pathology doing independent study on death investigations. "I had developed a strong interest in this field and I believed firmly that as a nurse I had a lot to offer it. I knew that since 1975, Dr. John Butts in Canada had used nurses to investigate deaths, but there was no place here in the States that I could fulfill my desire to practice."

Finally a position became available in the county where she lived. It was the first time a medical examiner system was being established here with adjoining metropolitan exam. "I met the criteria for the job and was hired, a duly authorized deputy of the chief medical examiner." The medical examiner had wanted to hire someone with a medical background, especially in psychiatry, and with an orientation to forensic science.

Virginia worked for eleven years in the field. Those in the local law enforcement felt sure she would fall flat on her face; as with any woman breaking into a male-centered job, Virginia had to constantly prove credibility. "We're trained differently than they are. We don't duplicate the same skills, but we complement each other skills. They view our lack of knowledge in one area that they excel in as being defunct, but they fail to take into consideration their lack of biomedical science knowledge, natural disease processes, trauma, medication, and our nursing interpersonal communication skills."

Despite their flack, the community supported her and appreciated her work with grieving families. Because of her abilities, problems for surviving families were greatly reduced.

As a death investigator, Virginia recognized the value of forensic practice in clinical nursing, a combination almost unheard of then. "No one teaches the student nurse how to identify crime victims, the signs and symptoms of abuse, wound character, gun-shot wounds, bite marks or documentation for med.-legal cases and courtroom testimony, but all these are crucial to understanding forensic nursing. I realized that if I wanted to teach this to nurses, I would have to get a masters degree in a field that had not yet existed."

Virginia wrote up the first masters degree program that would prepare a clinical nurse for the specialty. She approached Dr. Daniel Hughes, the dean in her home state university, the University of Texas at Arlington. He was interested from the beginning, but the crux was getting the curriculum committee to approve it. They were hesitant until a pathologist in Sweetwater, Texas, complimented them and pointed out the value of training nurses in the forensic arts. "And so the course was born."

The original focus was to prepare nurses for all events—death investigation, sexual abuse, criminalist, legal aspects, and expert-witness testimony, but espe-

268   Acknowledgments

cially to assist the forensic pathologist in the death investigation. Then she realized the challenge of clinical forensics: "We needed to expand into the twenty-first century and to develop relationships with other areas of forensic science. Nurses who are death investigators also need to be cross-trained as sexual assault examiners since the skills in investigating one can often help the other."

As a result of her work Virginia has presented the model of the clinical forensic nurse to the White House, explaining why forensic nursing is so important and why we need support.

Thanks to all those members of International Association of Forensic Nurses (IAFN) who helped with this book, many of whose names appear on the following pages.

A donation, based on the proceeds, will be made to the scholarship fund of IAFN, which will help forensic nursing research and students.

All of the cases here are actual cases discussed by members of IAFN. Some of the names of the nurses, participants, and locales have been changed to protect confidentiality and ethics, especially in cases that are still ongoing.

Thanks to the support and help of the following people, all of whom—mostly IAFN members—have contributed to the book. Also, thank you to my editor Ruth Cavin for being *so* patient and *so* caring and helpful in working on this book and in giving her time for such a worthy cause.

Denise Abbott

Eve Alexander

Gerri Anne

Kathy Bell

Mary Blair

Ann Burgess

Elizabeth Burki

Paul Clements Jr.

Gwendolyn Costello

Kathy Curtis

Connie Darnell

Joe Dominick

Patricia Duggan

Claudia Egan

Mary Jane Erickson

Diana Faugno

Jamie Ferrell

Marilyn Fisher

Marilyn Flynch

Pam Froncek

Marlene Galus

Barbara Gilbert

Sandra Goldstein

Sheryl Gordon

Nan Groth

Casey Harper

Carmen Henesy

Kim Henry

Sue Huber

Lee Johnson

Penni Joseph

Kris Karcher

Patty Kerr

Deborah Kilgore

Linda Klee

Melissa M. Krasko

Louanne Lawson

Linda Ledray

Gail Lenehan

Francine Likis

Jennifer Link

Virginia Lynch

Verlie Martin

Vicki Mayhall

Elena McAllister

Cynthia McCarthy

Marilyn McCarthy

John McPhail

Jacqueline McQay

Carolyn Meyer

Aubrin Miale

Vickie Milazzo

Stacy Lasseter Mitchell

Monica Mooney

Kim Moreno

Pat Morgan

Kathy Murphy

Barb Nelson

Sandi O'Brien

Georgia Pasqualone

Laura Reeves

Paul Reid

Pat Rouffel

Rene Rovere

Edith Rust

Barbara Salisburg

Ruth Seaburg

Barbara Sharer

A. J. Silvia

Robin Sparks

Pat Speck

Debbie Spicer

Sara Sullivan

Marilyn Swint

Julia Thompson

Donna Toohey

Lisa Tutice

Susan Webster

Rae Whooten

Celeste Williams

Deborah Williams

Kim Wilson

Susan Hiscoe Wisser

Pam Woods

Jean Zandra

And many others, some of whom asked not to be named.

My sincere apology for anyone inadvertently left off the list and to those I did not interview for this book due to lack of time and space.

Nearly all of these people are forensic nurses working in the field. Titles are not given, as I did not have access to all their titles and did not want to upset anyone by leaving titles out.

IAFN can be reached at 856-756-2425, www. IAFN.org, and the American Association of Forensic Science at 719-636-1100, P.O. Pox 699, Colorado Springs, CO 80901. For career information regarding forensic nurse training call 856-756-2425.

Bibliography

Aiken, M. M., "Documenting Sexual Assault in Prepubertal Girls," *American Journal of Maternal Child Nursing*, 15(3):176–77, May 1990.

———, "False Allegation: A Concept in the Context of Rape," *Journal of Psychosocial Nursing and Mental Health*, 31(11):15–20, Nov. 1993.

Aiken, M. M., and P. M. Speck, "Sexual Assault and Multiple Trauma: A Sexual Assault Nurse Examiners (SANE) Challenge," *Journal of Emergency Nursing*, 21(5):466–68, Oct. 1995.

American College of Emergency Physicians, "Management of the Patient with the Compliant of Sexual Assault," *Annals of Emergency Medicine*, 21:732, June 1992.

American Academy of Pediatrics Committee on Adolescents, "Sexual Assault and the Adolescent," *Pediatrics*, 94(5):761–65, Nov. 1994.

Barton, S., "Investigating Forensic Nursing," *Kansas Nurse*, 70(6):3–4, June 1995.

Bell, K. L., "The Tulsa Sexual Assault Nurse Examiner Program," *Oklahoma Nurse,* 40(3):16, 1995.

Besant-Matthews, P. *Gunshot and Stab Wounds: A Medical Examiner's View*, Barbara Clark Mims Associates, Dallas, Texas, 1993.

Brown, G. R., and D. K. Runyan, "Diagnosing Child Maltreatment," *North Carolina Medical Journal,* 55(9):404–408, Sept. 1994.

Buehler, J. Smith, E. Wallace, C. Heath, R. Kusiak, J. Herndon, "Unexplained Deaths in a Children's Hospital," *New England Journal of Medicine*, 313:211–16, 1985.

Burgess, A. W., and J. Fawcett, "The Comprehensive Sexual Assault Assessment Tool," *Nurse Practitioner*, 21(4):66, 71–72, 74–75, April 1996.

Burgess, A. W., W. Fehder, and C. Hartman, "Delayed Reporting of the Rape Victim," *Journal of Psychological Nursing and Mental Health*, 33(9):21–29, 1995.

Burgess, A. W., and L. L. Holstrom, "Rape Trauma Syndrome," *American Journal of Psychiatry*, 131:981–86, 1975.

———"Sexual Assault Signs and Symptoms," *Journal of Emergency Nursing*, 1(2):11–15, 1975.

Butts, J. D., "Injuries, Description, Documentation, Evidence Issues," *North Carolina Medical Journal*, 55(9):423–27, Sept. 1994.

Campbell, J., and D. Sheridan, "Emergency Nursing Interventions with Battered Women," *Journal of Emergency Nursing*, 15:12–17, 1989.

CDC Guidelines for Sexually Transmitted Diseases, 1993.

Committee on Quality Assessments: American College of Obstetrics and Gynecology, *Journal of Gynecology and Obstetrics,* 52(1):103–104, Jan. 1996.

Council on Scientific Affairs, American Medical Association, "Violence Against Women," *JAMA*, 267(23):3184–89, June 1992.

Cumming, M., "The Vision of a Nurse Coroner," *Journal of Psychosocial Nursing and Mental Health*, 33(5):29–33, 1995.

Davidson, J. R., D. C. Hughes, L. K. George, and D. G. Blazer, "The Association of Sexual Assault and Attempted Suicide Within the Community," *Archives of General Psychiatry*, 53(6):550–56, June 1996.

Davis, R., and J. Hooker, "If the Patient Is a Suspected Criminal," *American Journal of Nursing*, 79:1250–52, 1979.

Derman, S. G., and L. M. Peralta, "Postcoital Contraception: Present and Future Options," *Journal of Adolescent Health* 16(1):6–11, Jan. 1995.

Driscoll, K., "Search and Seizure in the Emergency Department," *Journal of Emergency Nursing*, 12:76–80, 1986.

Dupre, A., et al., "Sexual Assault," *Obstetrical and Gynecological Survey*, 48(9):640–48, 1983.

Epstein, J., and S. Langeheim, "The Criminal Justice and Community Response to Rape," *U.S. Department of Justice, National Institute of Justice*.

Frank, D., "The Perception of Self-esteem in Female Victims of Sexual Assault," *Florida Nurse*, 44(5):19, Feb. 1991.

Fulmer, T., S. Street, and K. J. Carr, "Abuse of the Elderly: Screening and Detection," *Journal of Emergency Nursing*, 10:131–40, 1984.

George, H., and M. Quaitrone, "Law and the Emergency Nurse Reporting Child Abuse," *Journal of Emergency Nursing*, 14:34–35, 1988.

Golden, G. S., "Use of Alternative Light Source, Illumination in Bite Mark Photography," *Journal of Forensic Science*, 39(3):815–23, May 1994.

Griffith, H., "Expert Nurse Witness," *Nursing BC*, 1:8, Jan. 1994.

Hampton, H., "Care of the Woman Who Has Been Raped," *New England Journal of Medicine*, 332(4):234–37, Jan. 1995.

Hofland, S., "Testifying in Court," *Clinical Nurse Specialist*, 4(4):212–14, 1990.

Howard, J., and M. Monhaut, "Behavioral Issues: Suicide by Vehicular Crash—Recognition and Early Intervention," *Journal of Emergency Nursing*, 14:230–33, 1988.

Hoyt, C., "Recognition and Collection of Evidence in the Clinical Setting,"

Hoyt, C., and K. Spangler, "Forensic Nursing Implications and the Forensic Autopsy," *Journal of Psychosocial Nursing*, 34:10, 24–27, 1996.

Hyden, P. W., and T. W. Gallagher, "Child Abuse Intervention in the Emergency Room," *Pediatric Clinics of North America*, 39(5):1053–81, Oct. 1992.

International Association of Forensic Nursing, "Standards of Practice for a Sexual Assault Nurse Examiner," P. Speck and IAFN SANE Council, 1996.

Jessee, S. A., "Recognition of Bite Marks in Child Abuse Cases," *Pediatric Dentistry*, 16(5):336–39, Sept. 1994.

Keating, S., and W. Allard, "What's in a Name? Medical Samples and Scientific Evidence in Sexual Assaults," *Journal of Medicine, Science and Law*, 34(3):187–201, 1994.

Kelley, S., "Physical Abuse of Children: Recognition and Reporting," *Journal of Emergency Nursing*, 14:44–47, 1988.

Kent-Wilkinson, A., "After the Crime, Before the Trial," *Canadian Nurse*, 89(11):23–26, June 1993.

Knickerbocker, M., "Protect the Victim, not the Criminal," *Nursing Life*, 5:26–29, 1985.

Koss, M., "Rape: Scope, Impact, Interventions and Public Policy Responses," *American Psychologist*, 48(10):1062–69, Oct. 1993.

Langlois, N. E., and G. A. Gresham, "The Aging of Bruises: A Review and Study of the Color Changes with Time," *Forensic Science International*, 50(2):227–38, Sept. 1991.

Laws, A., and J. M. Golding, "Sexual Assault History and Eating Disorder Symptoms Among White, Hispanic, and African-American Women and Men," *American Journal of Public Health*, 86(4):579–82, April 1996.

Layman, M. J., C. A. Gidycz, and S. J. Lynn, "Unacknowledged Versus Acknowledged Rape Victims: Situational Factors and Post-traumatic Stress," *Journal of Abnormal Psychology*, 105(1):124–34, Feb. 1996.

Ledray, L., "Counseling Rape Victims: The Nursing Challenge," *Perspectives in Psychiatric Care*, 26(2):21–27, 1990.

———, "Date Rape Drug Alert," *Journal of Emergency Nursing*, 22(1):80, Feb. 1996; *Journal of Public Health*, 86(4):579–82, April 1996.

———, "Rape or Self-injury?" *Journal of Emergency Nursing*, 20(2):88–90, April 1994.

———, "Sexual Assault Evidentiary Exam and Treatment Protocol," *Journal of Emergency Nursing*, 21(4):355–59, Aug. 1995.

———, "The Sexual Assault Examination: Overview and Lessons Learned in One Program," *Journal of Emergency Nursing*, 18(3):223–31, June 1992.

———, "Sexual Assault Nurse Clinician: An Emerging Area of Nursing Expertise," *AWHONNS*, 4(2):180–90, 1993.

———, "Sexual Assault Nurse Examiner Programs," *Journal of Emergency Nursing*, 22(5):460–65, Oct. 1996.

Lipscomb, G. H., D. Muram, P. M. Speck, and B. M. Mercer, "Male Victims of Sexual Assault," *Journal of the American Medical Association*, 267(22):3064–66, June 1992.

Lynch, V., "Biomedical Investigation as a Mental Health Nursing Role, in Lancaster," *Journal of Adult Psychiatric Nursing*, ed. 3. (Medical Examination Publishing, 1988.)

———, "Clinical Forensic Nursing: A New Perspective in the Management of Crime Victims from Trauma to Trial," *Critical Care Nurse Clinics of North America*, 7(3):489–507, Sept. 1995.

———, "Forensic Aspects of Health Care: New Roles, New Responsibilities," *Journal of Psychosocial Nursing and Mental Health*, 31(11), Nov. 1993.

———, "Forensic Nursing: Diversity in Education and Practice," *Journal of Psychosocial Nursing and Mental Health Services*, 31:11, 1993.

———, "Forensic Nursing: What's New?" *Journal of Psychosocial Nursing and Mental Health*, 33(9):6–8, Sept. 1995.

———, "Forensic Nursing in the Emergency Department: A New Role for the 1990s," *Critical Care Nursing Quarter*, 14:3, 1991.

———, "The Registered Nurse Functioning as an Investigator of Death," lecture.

———, "Role of the Forensic Nurse Specialists in the Identification of Sexual Assault Trauma," lecture.

MacFarlane, M., and P. Hawley, "Sexual Assault: Coping with Crisis," *Canadian Nurse*, 869(6):21–24, June 1993.

Malestic, S. L., "Fight Violence with Forensic Evidence," *RN* 58(1):30–32, Jan. 1993.

Marsh, T. O., "A Nurse's Guide to Sleuthing," *RN*, 41:48–50, August 1978.

Master, W. H., and V. E. Johnson. *Human Sexual Response*, 1966, NY.

McEwen, J., and P. Reilly, "A Review of State Legislation on DNA Forensic Data Banking," *American Journal of Human Genetics*, 54:941–58, Feb. 1994.

Merkin, L., and M. J. Smith, "A Community-based Model Providing Services for Deaf and Blind Victims of Sexual Assault and Domestic Violence," *Sexuality and Disability*, 13(2):97–106, Summer 1995.

Mittleman, R., H. Goldberg, and D. Waksman, "Preserving Evidence in the Emergency Department," *American Journal of Nursing*, 83:1652–56, 1983.

Muram, D., "Child Sexual Abuse," *Obstetrics and Gynecology*, 5:784–90, Dec. 1993.

Muram, D., K. Miller, and A. Culter, "Sexual Assault of the Elderly Victim," *Journal of Interpersonal Violence*, 7(1):70–76, March 1992.

National Victim Center and Crime Victim Research and Treatment Center, "Rape in America: A Report to the Nation," Washington, DC, 1992.

Norvell, M., G. Benrubi, and R. Thompson, "Investigation of Microtrauma After Sexual Intercourse," *Journal of Reproductive Medicine*, 29(4):269–71, April 1984.

O'Brien, C., "Medical and Forensic Examination by a Sexual Assault Nurse Examiner of a Seven-Year-Old Victim of Sexual Assault," *Journal of Emergency Nursing*, 18(3):199–204, June 1992.

Palmer, L., "The Impact of Child Sexual Abuse on the Children of Survivors," *Journal of Psychosocial Nursing and Mental Health Services*, 34(10):42–46, 1996.

Patel, H., M. Courtney, and M. Forester, "Colposcopy and Rape," *American Journal of Obstetrics and Gynecology*, 169(4):1334, April 1993.

Plumbo, M. A., "Clinical Practice Exchange. Delayed Reporting of Sexual Assault: Implications for Counseling," *Journal of Nurse Midwifery*, 21(4):355–59, Aug. 1995.

Robinson, K. *Forensic Nursing and Multidisciplinary Care of the Mentally Disordered*, London, 1999.

Saferstein, R. *Criminalistics: An Introduction to Forensic Science*, Prentice Hall, 1995, 5th ed.

Sklar, C., "Reportable Deaths," *Canadian Nurse*, 78:14–15, 1982.

Slaughter, L., and C. R. V. Brown, "Cervical Findings in Rape Victims," *American Journal of Obstetrics and Gynecology*, 164(2):528–29, 1991.

———, "Colposcopy to Establish Physical Findings in Rape Victims," *American Journal of Obstetrics and Gynecology*, 166:83–86, Jan. 1992.

Sloan J., A. Kellermann, D. Reay, et al., "Handgun Regulation, Crime, Assault and Homicide," *Nursing England Journal of Medicine*, (319):1256–62, 1988.

Smock, W., C. Ross, and F. Hamilton, "Clinical Forensic Medicine: How ED Physician Can Help with the Sleuthing," *American Health Consultants*, 5:1, 1994.

Speck, P. M., "20 Years of Community Service. Memphis Sexual Assault Resource Center," *Tennessee Nurse*, 58(2):15, 17–18, April 1995.

Standing Bear, Z. G., "Will the Vision Be Co-Opted," *Journal of Psychosocial Nursing*, 33:9, 59–64, 1995.

Stewart, C., "Nursing Management of Gunshot Wounds to the Head," *Journal of Neurosurgical Nursing*.

Thomas, M., and H. Tulsa Zachritz, "Sexual Assault Nurse Examiners (SANE) Program," *Journal of Oklahoma State Medical Association*, 86(6):284–86, June 1993.

Torress, J. E., and M. A. Riopelle, "History of Colposcope in the United States," *Obstetrics and Gynecology Clinics of North America*, 20(1):1–67, March 1993.

Turner, J., "Role of the ED Nurse in Health Care–based Hostage Incidents," *Journal of Emergency Nursing*, 10:40–45, 1984.

Ullman, S. E., and J. M. Siegel, "Victim-Offender: Relationship and Sexual Assault. Violence and Victims," 8(2):121–34, Summer 1993.

White, K., "Clinical and Medico-legal Considerations in the Management of Gunshot Wounds," *Critical Care Update*, 7:5–18, 1980.

Woolsey, S., "Support After Sudden Infant Death," *American Journal of Nursing*, 88:1348–55, 1998.

Young, W., et al., "Sexual Assault: Review of a National Model Protocol for Forensic Evaluation," *Obstetrics and Gynecology*, 80(5):878–83, Nov. 1992.